Rage Against Age

Charles E. Anderson, M.D., F.A.A.F.P.
Frank Covino, B.S., M.S.

Rage Against Age

Published in the United States by:
New Century Promotions
3711 Alta Loma Drive
Bonita, CA 91902
(800) 768-8484

Cover photo by Barbara Covino

ISBN 1-890035-14-9

10 9 8 7 6 5 4 3 2 1

Endorsements

"Dr. Anderson and Frank Covino have written a book based on a lifetime of clinical and firsthand experience. Their mission is to enhance the vitality and preservation of function of patients and colleagues. Dr. Anderson is listening to his patients and practicing thc Art of Medicine."

Steven Lamm, M.D.
Clinical Assistant Professor of Medicine, NYU
Author of *Younger at Last* and *The Virility Solution*

"*Rage Against Age* is a common sense approach to optimal health, utilizing diet, supplements, hormonal balancing, and exercise to achieve enhanced energy, vitality and longevity."

Ken Bock, M.D.
Author of *The Road to Immunity*
and *Natural Relief for Your Child's Asthma*

Dedications

My parents, Rose and Charles, who gave me the courage and tenacity to choose my life's path and passion in medicine despite numerous obstacles.

My godparents, Grace and Vincent, who have always been there for me and my family.

My wife, Amanda, my partner in all things; the wind beneath my wings.

Our children, Ryan and Samantha, who keep me going with their innocence, youth and perpetual growth.

Charles E. Anderson, M.D.

This gratifying effort is dedicated to:

My precious wife, Barbara, who sparked my rejuvenation the moment we met over 15 years ago. My principal motivation for aggressively fighting the aging process is to spend more active and productive time with her. Our only regret is that the information we reveal in these pages was not available to prolong the lives of our parents. Perhaps this information will enlighten my son and daughter, my sister and brothers, and their respective families.

Frank Covino

Disclaimer

Our book encourages its readers to take more personal responsibility for their health, but we affirm that seeking active health and longevity from exercise and nutritional supplementation should be done in cooperation with a qualified doctor. Wise physicians are becoming aware of the benefits derived from disease-preventive methods, like optimum nutrition, vitamin, mineral and anti-oxidant supplements, hormone replacement, and of course, exercise. These physicians refer to themselves as complementary physicians, practitioners of alternative therapies. Dr. Charles Anderson is a highly respected member of this medical community.

This book is in no way intended as a prescription for the reader. We are the first to admit that this is but one case history. You are unique. You have your own set of individual variations—physical, mental, and emotional. Only a doctor who knows, examines, and treats you can prescribe for you. For this reason, the authors and publishers of this book cannot take medical or legal responsibility for having the contents of this book considered a prescription for anyone. Consider the book as only a personal testimony of the authors, physical evidence of their own doctor/patient relationship, which followed twenty years of research and personal development by each of them in their quest for active health and longevity.

Acknowledgments

The Authors would also like to acknowledge and thank the following people, who proofread and critiqued this manuscript:

Amanda Anderson
Barbara Covino
Beth Friese
Master David Quinlan
Dr. Kelly Rybicki
Barbara and Gene Torvend
Grace Walsh

Many thanks to Carl Kunz for superb photography work.

Special thanks to Kelli Provost, our typist, who has redone this manuscript over and over again. Thank you, Tom, Gary, and Josh for arranging those late night sessions at Sugarbush Sports Center, and warm gratitude to the owner of the Powerhouse Gym in Bayside, New York for allowing me to drop in during my Mom visits at a generous cut rate. Thank you Joyce Standish for your editing. Thank you Charles Attal and Glenda Gasmen at New Century Promotions for all your support.

We cannot think of a better gift for each of you than this manuscript of truth. When you pass your hundredth birthday, strong, alert, and productive, please pass this information on to your closest friend, if they have not expired from self-inflicted disease and environmental pollution.

About the Authors

Dr. Charles E. Anderson, M.D., F.A.A.F.P.

A Hudson County, New Jersey emigrant to the Green Mountains of Vermont at the age of seventeen, cum laude graduate from St. Michael's College in Winooski, Dr. Charles Anderson earned his Medical Degree in 1971 at the University of Bologna Medical School in Bologna, Italy. His post-graduate residencies in Family Practice, Pediatrics and Allergies, included Wilson Memorial Hospital in Binghamton, New York, St. Vincent's Hospital of Worcester, Massachusetts, Children's Hospital of Boston, Massachusetts, and the Albany Medical Center of Albany, New York. He is a Fellow of the American Academy of Family Practice, the American College for Advancement in Medicine, the American Academy of Anti-Aging Medicine, and the Vermont State Medical Society.

For many years, Dr. Anderson was involved with the task of teaching medical students, interns, and residents within a hospital setting and private office-based practice. In the early 1980's, he was one of the first physicians in Vermont to work jointly in his practice with physician assistants and nurture their well-accepted role in the medical community. Through the years, Dr. Anderson has had great respect for the benefits of chiropractic medicine, and since the late 1970's, has had numerous chiropractic physicians working with him in his office for the overall benefit of his patients.

Dr. Anderson has had his own private practice for 25 years and has published numerous investigative articles in medical journals. Often called upon to lecture at medical seminars, he is quite comfortable before an audience, broadcasting his own medical radio talk show for four years on Saturday mornings, called "Health and Longevity." Dr. Anderson became actively involved in alternative therapies in 1986, prescribing nutritional changes, vitamin and mineral supplementation, and hormone replacement for his patients before resorting to drugs. His recommended regimens have been effective enough in many case histories for his patients to not have had to resort to drug prescription.

Dr. Anderson is approaching the age of 55, but looks and feels much younger due to his self-administration of supplements prescribed for his patients, plus his self-imposed active lifestyle with participatory interests, including horseback riding, downhill skiing, and karate. He has earned a second degree brown belt in Kempo and Kung Fu. Strength for his achievement in his chosen sports comes from periodic visits to weight-resistance health clubs, where he can isolate individual muscle development and avoid the problem of localized atrophy so common in lethargic men of his age. Co-author Frank Covino and his wife are prime examples of the efficacy of Dr. Anderson's complementary medicine and hormone replacement regimens. With supplements alone, he lowered Frank's cholesterol from 289 to 190 in three months and dropped Barbara Covino's cholesterol number from 337 to a remarkable 199 in two months. Both patients have changed their silhouettes dramatically. Dr. Anderson has probably increased their life expectancy. This complementary physician is constantly searching for natural substances, diet modifications, and physical therapy to replace traditional drug choices of mainstream medicine. He is a doctor who practices what he preaches, nurturing his patients with regimens that always begin with sincere motivation and patient/doctor dialogue. His co-author views Dr. Charles Anderson as a forerunner of 21st-century medicine.

Frank Covino—Artist, Author, Art Instructor

Frank Covino lives with his wife Barbara in a chalet at the foot of the challenging ski trail mountain known as Mt. Ellen in the Sugarbush Valley, Vermont ski resort. His first art book, *The Fine Art of Portraiture* (Van Nostrand Reinhold, 1970), was the result of seven years of research that earned him a Master's of Science degree in Art Teacher Education from Pratt Institute in New York City, summa cum laude. Following graduation, Frank taught the portrait and figure lessons for the Famous Artists School in Westport, Connecticut before opting to teach privately, forming his own Academy of Art in Fairfield County, Connecticut in 1962. Covino closed the doors to his Academy 25 years later to take his classical method to distant students. He presently conducts one-week workshops nationwide, visiting up to 30 cities a year, from Anchorage to Orlando. Since 1964, the artist has personally guided students through the completion of more than 17,500 paintings.

Two other art instruction books by the author include: *Discover Acrylics with Frank Covino* (Watson-Guptill, 1974) and *Controlled Painting* (Northlight, 1982). He has conducted numerous workshops around the country and has completed ten video tapes in his Art Education Series, which include the classical academic approach to painting with oils, sculpting with clay, and sketching with pastels.

Frank's portrait of singer Dinah Shore was unveiled during the popular national television show *20/20.* While the portrait received accolades, the artist's name was inconsiderately not mentioned. The portrait may be seen at the Mission Hills Country Club in Palm Springs. Reproductions of Covino's portrait have appeared on several billboards leading into the popular resort. He was commissioned to paint the last portrait of actress Gloria Swanson shortly before she passed away, and also one of the late popular singer Marvin Gaye, before his sudden departure. Several years ago, the World Wrestling Federation hired Covino to create the bronze, two-figure study for their heroic championship trophy, the "Slammy" award. A true follower of his Renaissance ancestors, the artist can create accurate realistic forms in any medium.

In November of 1995, the Louvre invited Covino to place 15 of his best students on the floor of the Paris Museum to copy Old Master paintings from the 17th, 18th, and 19th centuries. Frank took the toughest assignment upon himself, copying the difficult haunting image of *La Giaconda*, da Vinci's "Mona Lisa." His reproduction is incredibly accurate. You may view Frank's replication on his web site, www.portrait-art.com.

The author's avocation, since 1955, has been downhill ski instruction. Collaborating with renowned Olympic champion, Stein Eriksen, Covino produced a nationwide newspaper column in 1963 called, *Ski Tips* (King Features, 1963), and three instructional books, *Skiing Made Easy* (1971), *Skiers Digest* (1976), and *Downhill Skiing* (1979). Featured in the last two books is his singular experiencc skiing the challenging British Columbia mountain range called the Bugaboos, sponsored by Air Canada and the generosity of the famed Hans Gmoser. His uphill vehicle was a helicopter. His courageous wife was the photographer. From 1962 to 1972, Frank was a popular ski instructor at Sugarbush Valley, requested by many celebrities. Today, at 67, he can still be seen there conducting private lessons, admittedly a compulsive teacher.

Rage Against Age is the culmination of a manuscript begun by Covino in 1972, then titled *Active Longevity*. It was shelved for over 25 years, while the author aged, to give his conjecture credibility. Covino searched for a complementary physician who agreed with his opinions and could monitor his progress through his senior years. Dr. Anderson is his choice. We can all surely benefit from their collaboration.

Table of Contents

Foreword

Charles Anderson, M.D., F. A. A. F. P.

How often have you heard someone make a birthday wish that you live to be 100 and that they "hope to be around to celebrate it with you?" You have probably thought of this comment as nothing more than a good-humored toast or a hollow promise, but the truth is we should all aspire to live beyond 100 years. Science has demonstrated that we all have the capacity to live this length of time. The reason why few achieve this full life span is that most of us do not know how to stop the aging process, an accumulation of debilitating influences that make us vulnerable to disease, robbing us of our strength, our health, and ultimately, our full life expectancy. There are ways to intervene and interrupt this aging–disease–aging cycle. The concerned general public and some in the medical profession have come to realize that the most effective solution to aging, as with any disease, is prevention. For the first time in medical history, physicians and scientists are increasingly focused upon not just combating individual diseases but upon the entire process of aging, its specific causes, and preventive alternatives.

One form of aging is a cumulative destruction of weakened, undefended cells on a massive scale, leading to a regrettable and frightening global degeneration of our body and minds. That kind of aging occurs when our cells are permanently damaged by continual attacks from chemical particles called free radicals. These free radicals are infiltrating molecules that are missing an electron. They desperately try to snatch one from any of the other healthy molecules in our bodies. Free radicals careen out of control through our bodies, attacking our cells, turning our fats rancid, rusting our proteins, piercing our cell membranes, and corrupting the genetic DNA code until the cells become dysfunctional, give up, and die. Berkeley/UCLA researcher, Dr. Bruce Ames, has estimated that our cells are attacked by 10,000 free radicals a day. Nutritional supplements are effective defenders against this daily invasion, many available to you over the counter (OTC) with no required prescription. The anti-aging revolution is here, and the growing army of informed citizens is still open for enlistment. We urge you to read on and take charge of your Self.

It has taken scientists nearly a century to confirm the human need for anti-oxidants like vitamin C. History records indicate that approximately 200,000 British soldiers died from lack of this vitamin before it was even identified. Deficiency diseases of the centuries prior to ours, such as scurvy or beriberi, are not common health problems in America today, though. Rather, we have marginal nutrition associated with marginal physical conditioning as more likely the causes that age most people. For example, you may have enough vitamin C to protect you from scurvy, but not enough for optimal health and a vigorous immune system; you may have the physical strength to walk to your car, but not enough muscle or aerobic capacity to hike up a mountain or run on the beach.

In addition to anti-oxidants and sufficient exercise, research centers around the country, including Harvard, Stanford, and Johns Hopkins, are now recognizing the importance of supplementing our own age-depleted hormones, calling them super hormones. The roles that these hormones play and their supplementation are making it now possible, even as the years pass, for us to grow young and have bodies that are strong, healthy, and vigorous throughout our senior years. Some super hormones that we have personally tested with positive results are melatonin, DHEA, pregnenolone, testosterone, estrogen, progesterone, thyroid, and human growth hormone. You will read about our research and implementation shortly.

Although the irony of having great health and extensive longevity is that all the extra years come at the end, we can achieve these goals and arrive there in a healthy state of body and mind. Aging is as inevitable as death, but the rate at which aging characteristics occur is not necessarily correlated with chronological age. A flexible relationship exists, where inevitable aging can occur at variable rates of time. If everyone inevitably aged and deteriorated at the same rate, it would mean that all of us had been pre-programmed in the same way; this is not the case. We propose to show you methods with which you can control your own specific aging process.

Co-author Frank Covino's physical countenance is only one example that challenges the fallacy behind the concept of programmed debilitation and the inevitability of premature aging. Frank was the quintessential 95-pound weakling in his early teens, the smallest of the entire junior high school graduating class 1946. Participation in high school gymnastics and a set of iron barbells quickly changed his physical appearance, enabling him to endure the pressures of Korean War combat for which he enlisted. But his adopted program of nutritional supplements four decades ago, emphasizing anti-oxidants and his diet limitation of simple sugars and starches, all are responsible, I believe, for his currently active longevity. Frank will be seventy in 2001. Supplementation of precursors like DHEA, pregnenolone, Tribulus Terrestris, 19-Norandrostenedione, 19-Norandrostenediol, and the prostate protectors, Saw Palmetto and Pygeum, have elevated his formerly low testosterone to youthful levels, while Growth Hormone is regenerating his IGF-I. At 67, Frank was still teaching downhill skiing in the Green Mountains of Vermont. He has the strength of an Olympian athlete and he is but one of many patients who trust in the research and conjecture of complementary physicians.

We can change our lives and be masters of our destiny. We have the ability to approach our full life span with strong bodies and creative minds. Don't procrastinate. Take a wait-and-see attitude and you will encounter a paradox. If you wait too long, you will not be able to see because of the destruction brought about by macular degeneration and cataracts. Now is the time to take stock of yourself. *Rage Against Age!* Enjoy the "last of life", as Browning advises, "for which the first was made."

"Do not go gentle into that good night,

Old age should burn and rave at close of day;

Rage, rage against the dying of the light."

Dylan Thomas (1914-1963)
Do Not Go Gentle into That Good Night [1952]

Introduction

Your Invitation To Active Longevity

Frank Covino, B.S., M.S., A.T.E.

It is a black mark on the achievement records of parenthood that 22% of the young men who were drafted for service to our country during the Vietnam conflict failed their pre-induction examination for physical inadequacies. During the Korean War, our heavy causality list was fraught with names of young men who were injured or killed because of pre-induction physical limitations. Many of these men lost their lives simply because they could not run a few hundred yards. In either direction. One of us had the good fortune of being among the surviving enlisted men of that conflict, and I can testify that ours is not the only nation where physical conditioning has been added to the list of non-lucrative, non-hedonistic, and therefore, non-essential interests. "Able-bodied" men throughout the world have literally gone to pot. While the sarcasm and double entendre are offered with tongue in cheek, it is evident that the wave of puerile interest that has swept young men of all industrialized nations toward the shores of hallucinated euphoria, via the broad gamut of street drugs and recalcitrant Satanistic "music," has only added to their physical and mental disintegration, already begun by poor nutrition and lack of exercise. These aberrations of manhood, in the fullest sense of the word, are many of the fathers of today. Some are old enough to be grandfathers. Lethargic lifestyles have bred their contemporary teenagers who are in deplorable physical condition, and their projected life expectancy is shortening. Painfully aware of how this affects our national defense, the Pentagon recently launched Operation Be Fit (*N.Y. Times*, 1998) requiring 17- to 21-year-old men to be able to run 2 miles in 16 ½ minutes, perform 47 continuous sit-ups, and 35 non-stop push-ups in its Army of the millennium. Few high school seniors can pass this exam. Physical training is no longer mandatory in many of our schools. Since we are all products of heredity and environmental influence, what kind of picture can we paint of the fathers and sons of the future? Add to that depressing image paint from the currently powerful liberated woman's palette, and the portrait of tomorrow's man becomes an abstract distortion of the original product, stripped of so much of his masculine identity that he will be difficult to distinguish from the female of his species.

The contemporary label of unisex on the clothing, jewelry, and hair for today's "man" is a portent of the unnatural breed that the future awaits if someone does not take a stand against this perverse evolution! A popular song asks, "Where have all the flowers gone?" The flowers are here. It is the men who have gone. An interesting result of a return to natural order is that the more masculine a man's body looks, the better will be his chances for active longevity, just as the woman whose body is well-developed will probably live longer than her poorly conditioned neighbor, who will suffer through her late years with common old-age maladies. This book is not directed toward macho dominance over the fairer sex. Its purpose is to increase every reader's enthusiasm for life, to give man and woman the strength, health, and endurance necessary for them to function well beyond what statistics tell us is the average life expectancy.

Your body is a good barometer for your longevity potential. When is the last time you honestly evaluated its condition? Standing before a mirror with your mate, there should be an obvious difference between your silhouettes. The common silhouette prevalent among both sexes today respects no gender; from the head to the hips; it is the shape of a capital "A." Many men's suits are designed for this contemporary peculiarity. If your body falls into this category, you may be reasonably certain that only a miracle or accident of nature will allow you to see your eightieth birthday in good health. A 1998 report in the journal *Science* reveals 54% of American citizens to be heavier than is healthy, as their preponderance of weight is fat. This book can be the revelation that will change that torso of yours to a capital "V" and prolong your *active* years well beyond your one-hundredth birthday. We have noted active years in italics, because, if living beyond eighty means vegetating like the "retired" who migrate to the rocking chairs of Collins Avenue in Miami Beach, or like the stroke-prone condominium dwellers who populate other last- lap retirement communities, then the prospect of old age is certainly not an attractive one. If those poor misguided souls represent the only lifestyle available to us in our sunset years, it would be better to die young and be better looking corpses. Geriatrician Edward Bortz said it well in an interview with the editors of *Prevention Magazine*: "When a man retires from life, life retires from him." It depresses us to see that the poor nutrition habits and lack of exercise responsible for creating strange shapes among the walking dead in Miami Beach continue to characterize their lifestyles to the very end.

Every fast food restaurant is filled with diabetics, hypoglycemics, stroke and heart cases who continue to stuff themselves with sugar and starch in all their various forms. These oldsters avoid even mild exercise like the plague. Our apologies go to the Florida Chamber of Commerce for singling out their beautiful state as a case in point. We are very fond of Florida and, in fact, have enjoyed many vacations there. Certainly, every state has its share of rocking-chair corpses of people who have destroyed themselves with the same poor health habits mentioned, Vermont notwithstanding. In this country alone, more than 12 million people per day are sick enough to require medical care. It is just that they seem to form a monopoly along Miami Beach's Collins Avenue, as if someone designated that once-beautiful area as a nice place to die. The beach seems to cry for survival now, as the mammoth hotels which breach it cater to the strange suffering pilgrimage of senescents by providing the last word in Rococo pleasures, lest their guests miss some hedonistic satisfaction when their time has run out. The accent in typical retirement communities is on clothing (after all it "makes the man"), jewelry, big cars, and possessions (say it with hunched shoulders as you rub your hands together). If their money could only buy health.

Longevity with good health is for sale, but the rate of exchange has nothing to do with money. To pass us by, all the Grim Reaper asks from us is effort; daily physical effort; strenuous physical effort to keep our bodies functioning in the manner for which they were designed. He also asks that we use our minds in the accumulation of meaningful knowledge; the kind of knowledge that will permit us to be mentally and physically active in our late years. We must try to accumulate knowledge of: proper nutrition to fuel the active body, sociology and psychology, which will permit us to understand the people around us; our history, in order to anticipate the future which always reflects it; arts and crafts, which will permit us to contribute something beautiful to society in exchange for all that we take from it; and language, in order to communicate. Diversified "holistic" education is essential to the complete development of human potential.

This kind of education, for some, ends with a high school or college diploma. Graduation seems to be a license to give up all physical and mental effort. We become lazy spectators and vicarious adventurers, satisfying the natural needs of our bodies and minds with our eyes. We identify with basketball players or football heroes on TV and watch them move their bodies; we visit exotic places by viewing adventure films on TV or in theaters; and we even exercise our emotions through the feelings of others by viewing plays and dramatic movies which are directed specifically for that purpose. Our teenagers worship rock music stars for expressing in public the emotion that kids guard behind their grass-stoked stoic facades. Our attitude becomes, "Why should we do? That takes effort. We'd rather pay to watch someone else do." The difficulty with that kind of reasoning is that no one else will die for us, and unless we get off our fat-laden bottoms and start doing, our time on this earth will be short. In addition you can rest assured that the final years will be suffering ones.

Six out of ten of us who manage to survive and live beyond 60 will suffer from degenerative diseases like heart trouble, high blood pressure, hardening of the arteries, osteoporosis, diabetes or hypoglycemia. These are conditions that can be prevented by proper nutrition and sensible exercise. The President's Council on Physical Fitness has advised: "Exercise, of course, cannot stop a person from getting older, but when properly applied can retard the aging process; it also adds vigor to living throughout life." Some forms of cancer can even be avoided, if we use our intelligence and give up destructive habits like the foolish practice of smoking. Even the area in which you live is a matter of choice. Some of you live in an urban environment where the local weather forecaster frequently labels the air quality as "unacceptable." Is the high income you earn in that filthy city worth shortening your life? What about the lives of those who depend on you? It is truly a question of values.

The average healthy life expectancy is getting shorter in our country, as it is in most industrialized societies, largely due to cardiovascular diseases. Our nation ranked among the first five countries of the world in the race against premature aging and death in 1930. We slumped to 51st place in 1978. Some improvement has occurred since then because of the anti-smoking campaign resulting from Framingham research, but the population of weak senescents is growing, and the future looks bleak if more Americans do not change their sedentary, gluttonous, hedonistic, and unknowingly self-destructive lifestyles.

The Framingham Heart Study solicited 5,209 local volunteers between the ages of 30 and 60 for epidemiological analysis. Of that group, 1,300 are still alive and under close scrutiny. Epidemiologists are observers, not practicing therapists. Their findings clearly point to correlations, providing neither specific cause nor even conjecture. But their studies "often provide the first clues to the causes of disease," according to deputy director, Dr. Peter Savage of the National Heart, Lung and Blood Institute. "It's only when we've developed strong clues to the mechanism of disease that we can start to design clinical trials to test ways of treating that disease."

Saturated fat (fat that solidifies at room temperature), i.e., butter and transfatty-acids (solidified by hydrogenation), i.e., margarine, were observed to be frequently ingested by the Framingham participants with high cholesterol counts; hence, the fat-phobic mania prevalent today. When the study began, most doctors thought smoking to be a harmless leisure activity, and some even endorsed cigarette brands. Many owned stock in tobacco companies. In 1948, the American Medical Association (AMA) refused to condemn the practice. The Framingham studies printed a direct correlation between smoking, lack of exercise, and heart disease, while many doctors at the beginning of the study were certain that exercise caused heart attacks rather than prevented them. We owe a great deal to the Framingham reports which have helped us take a giant step toward preserving health in our senior years.

It may be time for an honest evaluation of yourself in a full-length mirror, devoid of the three-hundred-dollar suit and fancy shoes which might impress your secretary, but which do nothing for your life-sustaining cardiovascular system (nor do they nourish your dormant muscles that are being choked with fat). There seems to be a direct correlation between the amount of money spent on clothing, jewelry, and colognes and the poor physical condition of the spender. You might think you are hiding your inadequacies with those surface embellishments, like a woman hides her poorly developed figure with caftans and blousy dresses. The fact is you are really kidding only yourself, and you might be headed for an early and unpleasant forced retirement. Atherosclerosis, heart attacks, and strokes are responsible for the termination of 10% of the work force in any civilized country at the age of 55. What should be the years of middle age have become the years of old age, not by any fluke of nature, but because of the stupidity of man and woman, exhibited in their lack of education and their distorted standards of values.

The doctor, seen frequently as a respectable member of the family and the hallowed M.D. in whom you place all of your trust to cure your various maladies, is probably not in much better shape than you. His profession, in fact, heads the list of occupations with a high mortality rate. More doctors die before age 65 than do men in any other profession. As late as 1965, the AMA refused to label smoking as bad for your health. Doctors specialize in pathologies; they are paid to recognize and treat diseases and physiological malfunctions. Few physicians are schooled in nutrition and health maintenance. When it comes to the prevention of premature aging through proper nutrition and exercise, many medical men know less than the average patient. You could say that the mainstream medical profession satisfies our diagnostic and curative needs, and for that they are indispensable, whereas complementary physicians, nutritionists and qualified physical culturists share their knowledge of how to avoid disease and physiological malfunctions with sound programs of nutrition and exercise that are preventive. Dr. Anderson is one of these avant-garde physicians. If more of us knew how to care for our health properly, doctors would have fewer patients. I do not mean to take a cheap shot at the profession in which I have some good health-conscious friends, but I have met so many other doctors who are disturbingly uninformed in the fields of nutrition and exercise, sciences which deal with prevention of the maladies for which they are constantly seeking cures. Some of these are in disgraceful physical condition and some are even drug dependent; as are many nurses.

I can remember many visits to our "family doctor" when I was a child. His obesity did not seem to bother my parents. Doctors were expected to look portly, a Victorian mark of affluence. He assisted mom in my delivery and had the most patients in his neighborhood. He also wore an expensive suit and had a penchant for prescribing mineral oil and enemas for many illnesses. His obesity finally killed him. Atherosclerosis. Or maybe it was his cigarettes. A steady habit of his prescribed mineral oil treatment might have killed some of his patients. Slowly, like small doses of arsenic. This oil cannot be digested. What it can, and does do, on its way to the intestines is captivate and deplete vital vitamins like A, D, E, and K. Medical journals have since warned physicians against the use of this popular, but degenerative, form of laxative. Of more concern to me than the possibility of misguided medical cures is the curious deprecation by some doctors of sensible preventive maintenance measures like the taking of vitamin supplements, despite scientific evidence of the efficacy in disease prevention. Supplemental vitamins are a vital necessity today, when valuable nutrients have been processed out of such common foods as white bread and flour products, but Orthomolecular Nutrition is not yet recognized as a science. The medical profession has always been slow to accept preventive or curative remedies that have no scientific history. Back-woods Vermonters have been treating heart trouble with an herb called "fox glove" for well over a century; it was discredited by the medical profession for years as having no scientific basis, but later accepted by them and renamed Digitalis only after its repeatedly successful results offered no alternative. Now, the drug is widely prescribed for heart conditions, limited to small doses, and has been successful in alleviating the symptoms of many heart malfunctions. Similar success in the treatment and prevention of many diseases by the use of vitamin and concentrated natural food supplements has still only impressed a small percentage of our nation's doctors, and that could have a direct bearing upon their own high mortality rate.

Professional men, with doctors up front, die of hardening of the arteries at a rate that is three and one-half times greater than that of unskilled workers, whose occupations require physical effort, like farmers, miners, and laborers. This statistic indicates that the skilled or highly educated are not necessarily the most intelligent when it comes to personal health maintenance. Apparently, the more sedentary an occupation is, the less chance an individual has of achieving active longevity. This suspicion has aroused the interest of one of your authors, since he is a professional involved in, besides the avocations of writing and physical culture, the lethargic business of producing art. I've been an oil painter and sculptor for over 30 years and have been teaching those crafts since 1962. Unlike other professional men in my field, however, I have not dedicated all my time and energies to art, and therein, may lie one of the explanations of good health and strength I have maintained as I approach the age of 70.

There is a history of other artists who attained active longevity because of their diversified interests which included strenuous exercise of some sort. In the era where the average age for dying was well below 40, the century of the Renaissance, master artists like Titian were living and producing art for as long as a century. Young and handsome Raphael was an exception, but we can guess that his unfortunately early departure may have been the result of his promiscuity, like that of the poor male giraffe who was mated to a dozen females at a well-known zoo recently in an effort to propagate the species. The giraffe made a heroic effort, setting a record in the number of his amorous climaxes, then unexpectedly died. Smiling. Fortunately, he did become a father. We do not know whether Raphael was as successful, but he did die early from a very popular disease. Michelangelo, though, was an octogenarian, productive to the last year of his life, and Leonardo da Vinci was another artist whose life doubled the average lifespan of his era. We know much of the phenomenal amount of significant achievements by both of these creative giants and, unfortunately, little about their nutritional habits. We can assume, though, that only a man of great strength and endurance could hack away as many chunks of hard Carrara marble as Michelangelo, and Vasari tells us that the genius of all ages, Leonardo, was strong enough to bend open a horseshoe with his bare hands. That kind of power can only be developed over a long period of time from strenuous exercise against heavy resistance. Da Vinci must have "worked out." No one is born strong. Can we not deduce that there is a direct relationship between hard manual labor and active longevity? Let's face it, we must move the body or it will decay, just as the mind will degenerate from lack of use. The National Adult Fitness survey, as reported by Dr. Robert Atkins on a 1999 TV informercial, claims that 45% of all adults in America engage in no physical exercise at all. Among those who do exercise, a great many reserve contact activity for weekends or for their annual two-week vacations. These part-time athletes are prime candidates for heart attacks and cerebral strokes. Weekend warriors.

A prominent New York dentist booked a weekend at our bed and breakfast for skiers a few years ago to learn how to ski. His companion assured us that the 50-year-old man was in great shape. "He's a biker," she claimed, "and he plays tennis, too." What she did not say was that these were only weekend activities. The rest of the doctor's time was spent with dentistry and Wall Street investments that had moved him up the ranks of success to the coveted status of millionaire. The night before his first ski lesson, he boasted about his biking achievements and assured me that he would be a rapid learner. In deference to Shakespeare, I refrained from saying, "...doth 'boast' too much, methinks."

Experience teaching over 6,000 skiers has taught me to not take a novice to the top of a hill until they first have learned the mechanics of a turn on flat ground. We usually begin lesson one at the bottom of the slope, climbing a little higher after each successful turn, for a slightly longer run. Ten steps of climbing thoroughly exhausted the "athletic" doctor. From beet-red, his face turned pale-blue, as sweat poured from his brow. "That's enough climbing," he insisted. "Take me up on the lift." "You're not ready for the lift," I advised. "You haven't learned to turn." Try as I did, no reason would convince the arrogant doctor that he was not ready for the beginner slope. He finally agreed that if I took him up and he was too frightened to ski down, he would take off his skis and walk down the side of the slope, while I skied down, carrying his equipment.

That the doctor was frightened is an understatement. Looking down from the top, he trembled with fear. His knees collapsed and he sat, staring downhill with bulging eyes. "Stay there a moment," I advised. "Watch me carefully as I demonstrate a turn in slow motion. Relax. Enjoy the sunshine and soft snow cushion." I talked through several demonstrations, waiting for signs of calm, but the doc's face was still pale-blue and the fear would not subside. "Take them off," I pleaded. "Walk down the side of the trail. I'll take your skis." This time, he welcomed my advice. More than fear was taking place, but I never anticipated what would follow.

At the bottom of the slope, I hammered the tails of the doctor's skis deep into the powder and watched his slow descent. Stabilized by his ski poles, he took what seemed like forever, but finally reached the flat. He looked gray. The ski lodge and warm fireplace beckoned, a few hundred yards away. Doc never made it. He dropped and never took another breath. No amount of CPR, administered for nearly an hour, could revive him.

I once read with compassion a revealing article in a Florida newspaper titled "A Doctor's Heart, an M.D.'s unflinching account of how he nearly lost his life—and then found it" by Dr. Jaswant Singh Pannu. Dr. Pannu was a practicing physician in Lauderdale Lakes, Florida, who suffered a heart attack Thanksgiving Day of 1976, which manifested itself as a complete blockage of his right coronary artery. His report is not medically oriented, but rather, is an emotional account designed to put the reader in touch with the fears and anticipations that a man might experience in the face of such a near-fatal infarction. The report begins with the doctor's surprise that he should have fallen prey to America's No. 1 disease when he had enjoyed "perfect health for a man of 42, exercising regularly, and showing no signs of serious physical problems." We were determined to scrutinize his manuscript to see if it included any clues to his cardiovascular disease susceptibility.

Early in the diary, recording the events on the day of the attack, is an account of the type of exercise in which the doctor engaged. He speaks of playing tennis. Since a doctor's work schedule is a busy one, we suspect that this was a weekend activity, perhaps on one day out of the week. Moreover, he was specifically playing doubles, teaming up with his partner, a cardiologist. He boasts that they "had an easy time with our opponents." The match was followed by a game of backgammon, which the doctor also lets us know he won. It was at that moment of victory that the first symptoms hit: hot and cold flashes, a pain in the left arm, a "knot in the breastbone."

Doctors generally agree that exercise is needed to regulate the blood chemistry, especially when we follow the average contemporary diet of excessive saturated fat, starch and sugar consumption, characteristic of our patronage of thousands of fast food conveniences. Statistics have also indicated that heart and circulatory problems may result from sporadic and short exercise periods, particularly when those brief moments of stress are not approached gradually with a related warm-up period. Weekend tennis is one sporadic sport that illustrates this type of unfavorable form of exercise, particularly when there are four players who make the moments of individual stress even more sporadic. Golf, where walking has been replaced by the comfort of the cart and the 19th hole with its attendant martini as the motivation for participation, is another sport that can be a slow killer. Winning is apparently an important motivation of weekend sportsmen like Dr. Pannu. He probably would not take part in a game or form of exercise which did not present the challenge of conquest. Such motivation can exhaust the adrenals with sudden stress in meeting the demand for excessive insulin secretion, and their collapse can create high blood pressure, heart attack, hardening of the arteries, kidney disease, and other infections which Dr. Hans Selye attributes to the "stress adaption syndrome." Dr. Selye was director of the Institute of Experimental Medicine and Surgery at the University of Montreal when his experiments revealed stress as a primary cause of premature aging and disease. We will speak more of Dr. Selye's work in a later chapter.

No heart in good condition can be damaged by regular exercise. Your cardiovascular system can actually be augmented, and thus, ameliorated, by progressive exercise which demands stress that is continuous over a sustained period of time. Such exercise, with progressive weight- resistance training leading the list of effective forms, awakens dormant muscle fibers which require their own blood supply in addition to that system with which your body has been previously functioning. In effect, you can create your own bypass system, which, incidentally, is the surgical alternative that saved the life of Dr. Pannu. In his case, a vein was borrowed from another area and hooked onto the artery just beyond the constriction to permit his blood to flow to the heart.

A second clue to the mystery of how a man of self-presumed "perfect health" could contract arterial blockage can be found recorded on the eighth day of his diary. Dr. Pannu writes: "Later, I did something else which made me feel good. I asked a friend to sneak me a Burger King 'Whopper' because I couldn't stand the hospital's food. He did it, and I thoroughly enjoyed the meal."

Granting Dr. Pannu's good sense to reject the hospital food, which is often notoriously high in starch and refined sugar, his substitution of a white bread sandwich fast food equally high in starch and processed carbohydrates, and doubly offensive in its grease and high animal fat content, was an indication of the doctor's poor nutritional education and quite possibly might be a clue to his arterial blockage. Dr. Pannu's bypass surgery was completed on January 28, 1977. The operation was successful, and he returned to his previous life style. "My tennis game is better than ever" was the closing statement of his report.

Before we lose all our readers who are tennis buffs, and that probably would be a considerable number considering the growing popularity of the sport, let us qualify our criticism of Dr. Pannu's choice of exercise by assuring you that it is only directed at professional people whose occupations require no physical effort for the bulk of the entire week. Like the weekend bicycling dentist. Exercises requiring sudden effort, like tennis, handball, baseball, football, all contact sports, do not promote cardiovascular health and in fact, challenge the cardiovascular and adrenal systems with sudden severe strain. These sports can be engaged in regularly by athletes who already have developed cardiovascular immunization (yes, it is possible), but certainly should not be occasionally practiced by office workers who lead a life of lethargy for five days a week and then tax their cardiovascular systems with such competitive sports on their days of off. Cardiovascular health-promoting sports include jogging, cross-country skiing, swimming, biking, and the repetitive type of progressive weight-resistance exercise, such as will be demonstrated in this book, for strength, shape, and endurance. Is it not curious that each of these health-promoting sports has no stressful prerequisite of *conquest* as its motivation? If you cannot take part in exercise without having victory as a goal, you have serious psychological problems. The only victory you will score in these healthy sports is the sure conquest of atherosclerosis, heart malfunctions and strokes. It is a question of values as to whether you consider these fatal opponents as significant as your tennis or golf adversaries.

Do not worry about training with weights if you have a tendency toward high blood pressure, unless your condition is serious enough to require medical treatment; in that case, by all means consult with your doctor before beginning a new exercise program. Just be certain to choose a doctor whose own physical appearance and vigor mark his adequate knowledge of sound nutrition and exercise. Proper weight-resistance training and diet can normalize your blood pressure.

Heart attacks and cerebral strokes are caused by arterial blockage. The plaque that accumulates on the inside walls of arteries and eventually blocks circulation of blood is caused by excessive fatty foods, the ingestion of too much refined carbohydrates or sugar, and/or cigarette smoking. It has been proven that the arteries of athletes who engage in cardiovascular health-promoting sports, such as we have listed, have been found to be much larger in diameter than those of the average man. By enlarging the diameter of your own arteries, it is certainly possible to achieve cardiovascular immunization. If you think that it is more important than a weekend of 6-loves, then read on.

An autopsy was performed upon Finnish marathon runner Paavo Nurmi, a known sugar and junk food addict, after he willed his body to medical science and accommodated us by dying much sooner than he should have. The results shocked the medical profession when they revealed his coronary arteries were three times the diameter of other men his weight and height who were less active. More significant is evidence that followed, which showed that the cholesterol deposits which hugged the inside walls of the enlarged arteries of this athlete with poor nutrition habits was sufficient in quantity to kill three average men. Only the enlarged diameter of Nurmi's arteries permitted adequate circulation of blood and oxygen, and thus life, whereas the arteries of non-athletes with the same amount of cholesterol would have suffered fatal constriction years before. Dr. Clement G. Martin assured us, in his 1963 book, *How to Live To Be 100*: "No one has ever been able to prove the occurrence of a heart attack in an athlete–in condition–<u>at any age</u> (athletes out of condition are in the same boat with the rest of us, of course)." There is now no doubt that cardiovascular immunization is possible by following a systematized program of progressive exercise designed to expand the amount of oxygen your cardiovascular system uses, as it steps up the activity of the heart. This book will provide such a program for you.

Before rebuilding your body and discovering the magnificent potential you have for muscular development and cardiovascular amelioration, we will look into some of the things that cause premature aging and discuss nutritional alternatives that are available to you to slow down the process of deterioration. We have no prescription for eternal life, but we know that we can prolong your life expectancy, if by nothing else, by simply adjusting your weight and exchanging your fat for functional muscle. One percent of your life expectancy may be deducted for each pound you are "overweight." About half the number of all males over 35 are 10% or more over their optimum body weight, and their excess is fat, not muscle; double that percentage for women. If too much weight is not your problem, your neurotic behavior and low energy level can still be a result of poor nutrition or lack of exercise. A few adjustments in your diet and your lethargic life style can help you to reach a later age in an active, and hopefully, productive condition. You will feel the difference, your friends will notice the difference, and society will profit from your newly acquired vital energies which will give you the capacity to be a significant contributor.

Your fountain of youth is only as far away as the pages of this book; someone has led you to the fountain, but no one can make you drink. If you are past 30, you have already learned that your chosen lifestyle has shaped the condition in which you are, and that pattern has been influenced by what you have learned, from reading, observing, and from practice, followed by your personally gratifying results. That gratification was affected by pleasure if you are a hedonist, or by pain if you are a masochist. In either case, we are all pragmatists, and even the least educated among us is the designer of his own fate, genetics and environmental influences notwithstanding. The choice is yours. You may read and discard what you have read as you might habitually dispose of the conjecture of "another health freak"; or read, take a close look at yourself, and choose to not change your self-satisfactory direction; or you might read, compare and use the information in these pages to adjust your life style after a reasonable amount of time has passed for your honest evaluation of its efficacy. It is with the hope that you will choose the latter direction that we are about to make this effort.

The basic goals of this book are to awaken and tone your dormant muscles, which may have been neglected for years, to ameliorate the condition of your heart, your lungs, your blood vessels and vital organs, to increase your energy level and maintain one which will increase your productivity and promote a zest for living, to challenge your dietary habits and provide a nutritional program that will revitalize and add years to your life. This zest will give you the strength, endurance and knowledge necessary to deter the inevitable aging process. While our principal motive will be to increase your internal efficiency, external benefits you will derive from adherence to the programs advised in this book will include a noticeable improvement in your physical appearance, more youthful vigor and enthusiasm, and, most probably, a happier and more gregarious disposition. This change in personality will follow your newly acquired sense of self-preservation and confidence, especially when you compare your new self with people your own age who have not been so enlightened.

If veterans who served in the Korean conflict of 1950-1953 were permitted a rebuttal against revisionist history, designed by the liberal guardians of our nation's youth, General Douglas MacArthur would be presented as a great leader. The general would not only have led us to victory against the communist Chinese were it not for an impulsive, naive President, but his Machiavellian insight would have affirmed the strength of democracy and most assuredly have prevented the Vietnam War that was to follow. Wise men respect the motivations and inspirations behind the wisdom of our great leaders. The indefatigable nature of General MacArthur may be revealed in the framed message that he hung over every new desk in his travels:

> "Youth is not a time of life—it is a state of mind. Nobody grows old merely by living a number of years; people grow old only by deserting their ideals. Years wrinkle the skin, but to give up enthusiasm wrinkles the soul. Worry, doubt, self-distrust, fear and despair—these are the long, long years that bow the head and turn the growing spirit back to dust.
>
> Whether seventy or sixteen, there is in every being's heart the love of wonder, the sweet amazement at the stars and the star-like things and thoughts, the undaunted challenge of events, the unfailing childlike appetite for what next, and the joy and the game of life.
>
> You are as young as your faith, as old as your doubt, as young as your self-confidence, as old as your fear, as young as your hope, as old as your despair." —Author Unknown

Other authors and publishers who have influenced our thinking, and whose books would serve as supportive conjecture to the advice presented in the pages that follow, are (in alphabetical order), Dr. Paavo Airola, Dr. Robert Atkins, Dr. Abram Hoffer, Dr. Hans J. Kugler, Dr. Clement G. Martin, Richard A. Passwater, Dr. Ivan Popov, Morton Walker, and Dr. Roger J. Williams, physical culturists Jack LaLanne, Dr. Laurence E. Morehouse, Bill Phillips, and Joe Weider, and nutritionists Adelle Davis, Dr. Carlton Fredericks, and Gayelord Hauser. I should also thank the editors of *Prevention Magazine* for providing a wealth of information on preventive maintenance for longevity. You could say that this book is a compendium of educative treatises on the subjects of nutrition, exercise, and longevity, which is offered with complete confidence and in good faith, as the pragmatic education has performed miracles for us and for our families.

Your author became seriously interested in nutrition and exercise when his father, a great athlete up to the age of 40, was hit with a fatal stroke. He had been sufficiently warned by his doctor to give up the self-destructive habit of smoking 10 years prior to his demise, but Dad was addicted. Coupled with lack of daily exercise (he gave it up completely), the habit of smoking constricted his coronary arteries and for the last five years of his life, he functioned as a partially coherent vegetable in the care of his loving and dedicated wife, Katerina. My Dad was only a few years past 60 when he died, what should have been the years of his middle age. If someone in your family has been similarly afflicted, I am certain that you do not wish to follow the same pathetic path. The authors of this book both exercise and select cautiously the foods they eat. The changes experienced in our physical development, energy level, and productivity are astounding, and we want to share them with you.

As this is a confidential report from one author who holds no medical degree but is physically fit as he approaches the age of 70, and one with a medical degree who is well-schooled in disease prevention, it is hoped that it will be used as a primer for other pragmatics. We have no products to sell. This book is only our personal testimonial. You are expected to examine the health program and take a position, affirmative or negative, but we ask that you consider how your decision will affect your own life. Our first suggestion you have already read twice: Look in a full-length mirror, naked, for an honest evaluation. Use a hand mirror also to get a good view of the rear which you never see. We do not have to tell you what to look for. You might even pass this first test; perhaps there are no rolls of dripping fat; maybe your waist is smaller than your chest; possibly your calf and flexed biceps do measure the same classical ideal proportion; your posture might be exemplary; on the surface you just might pass as well-developed. Now, how about function? What is your energy level? Can you run up ten flights of stairs without bursting your heart? In how many minutes can you jog five miles? Could you ski an expert ski trail non-stop? What is your resting heart rate? Is your libido a fond memory? How about your productivity; for what purpose do you exist?

You are what you look like when stark-naked. Your physical countenance is a result of your diet plus how you are using your body. You are also what you have produced, whether those accomplishments have been as world-stirring as the works of Leonardo da Vinci or as noble and significant as planting a tree. Your diet and physical activities have shaped the body you possess. Your productivity is the justification of your existence. Muscular development alone will not deter the aging process. You might have to adjust your eating habits. Biological deterioration takes place in every individual and is the direct cause of many fatal diseases. Such deterioration can cause the termination we call "death from old-age," but no one has every really died of old age. "Death by natural causes" usually means that a vital organ has deteriorated ahead of the other vital organs in the body which were dependent upon it for optimum performance. Improper nutrition can cause this deleterious effect. You can delay the process by feeding yourself properly. We will discuss some of the experiments, conjecture, and conclusions that have been offered on this subject by reputable men and women in the field of nutrition and Orthomolecular Medicine, the science of healing with nutrition therapy, as defined by Dr. Abram Hoffer. Stress is another important factor that contributes significantly to the aging process. You need to know the forms from which it manifests itself and look into authoritative conjecture and scientific evidence that indicate the changes you might need to make in your lifestyle.

At no time in this book will you read dogmatic statements that we present as irrefutable, for, in the final analysis, we are all individuals who have been subject to a myriad of hereditary and environmental influences. No single cure can possibly apply to everyone. The suggestions we make are motivated by the experiments we have performed upon ourselves and numerous patients and clients, after reading the same variety of thoughts which we are about to pass on to you. The effectiveness of such a prescription is dependent upon your own response. It is advised that you take a complete physical examination before trying any of our directions toward self-improvement and that you show this book to your physician to assure yourself that the advice presented can do you no harm. All we ask is that you choose a doctor whose own physical health matches his intellectual capacities. Your doctor, and in fact, every person with whom you come into contact in your lifetime, is an influential factor in your environment. It is a wise man who chooses the characters of that environment cautiously. You have been the designer of your own unique self, but your choices in that development were influenced by your environment and, of course, by heredity. You cannot change your heredity factors, but you can and should be in control of the factors of your environmental influence which most assuredly contribute to your longevity potential. Environmental influences include books you have read, like this one. If you are not satisfied with your present image, it is not too late to march to a different drummer. You have nothing to lose but your life.

A body in good health is the principal tool for the creative expression of the mind. A body in decay makes an invalid of the mind. Look about you and you will see many invalids in body and mind, excuses for human beings who trudge from their hated forms of employment home to their throne before the boob-tube, where they can slouch and stuff their misshapen bodies with greasy, fattening foods, alcoholic drinks, and empty calories, until years of physical inactivity and malnutrition makes them wards of the state or burdens upon surviving members of their family. Perhaps you are becoming one of these walking dead. It is not too late. You are searching for guidance or you would not have opened this book.

It was such a quest that led me to the co-author of this book, Dr. Charles Anderson. My original manuscript began in 1972 and was titled, *Active Longevity*. I had become proficient enough to teach in two fields, classical academic art and the exhilarating sport of downhill skiing. Adult students attending my classes led me to believe that the physical condition of men and women in the United States was deplorable, largely due to lack of physical activity beyond the age of 20. My professional status as a skier demanded fitness from continuous physical effort between winter seasons and frequent visits to gymnasiums that provided weights for progressive resistance training kept me physically fit. "If the aging process is the programmed debilitation of cells," I theorized, "what better way to stay ahead of this impending deterioration than to build muscle, awakening dormant cells and creating a whole new venal system to transport blood and re-nourish my heart?" My theory seemed to have added benefits apart from maintaining a "V" shape, while my peers gradually succumbed to an "A" or an "O", as my energy level was high and my brain was lucid enough to produce several books for the art and ski industries. My chosen nutritional regimen was influenced by the book, *Diet Revolution* by Dr. Robert Atkins; I became his disciple.

The manuscript was shelved for 30 years, however, as it needed a healthy "senior citizen" author to have any credibility. Since I lacked medical doctor credentials, an authoritative M.D. partnership was indicated. Dr. Atkins was a six-hour drive away from our Vermont home, but his office highly recommended Dr. Anderson, whose office is in Essex, Vermont, as a knowledgeable practitioner of "complementary medicine," a euphemism for the courageous doctors who keep up to date with drug-alternative therapy and holistic patient analysis. Dr. Anderson is a physically fit, athletic 55-year-old, with a computer-comparable brain that has retained volumes of prophylactic prescriptions, drug-free, for the amelioration and defeat of many forms of age-related illnesses. He was startled by my physical condition, when he read the dossier listing my age. Although I sported a beer gut, the rest of my body was strong. When I asked for advice to prolong active longevity, Dr. Anderson quipped that I had apparently achieved it. He asked if I worked out with weights. Despite my outwardly strong physical countenance, Dr. Anderson's examination of my blood indicated a low testosterone count and a high cholesterol number that previous doctors had proclaimed "normal for my age." After lowering that cholesterol count over 100 points in three months with vitamin supplements and increased aerobic activity, Dr. Anderson and I decided to collaborate in the writing of this book for the benefit of pragmatic readers who take a good look at the physical countenance of' authors and doctors before following their prescriptions.

No prescriptions are provided for you in this book, however, as each of you has a personal history of nutrition and physical condition that is singular. The authors will only use themselves as examples. You will read about theories that we have tested personally and you will witness, by photographs, the results. It is suggested that you confer with an M.D. who practices complementary medicine before trying any of the therapies mentioned in this book. You may find your doctor the same way I found Dr. Anderson, by writing or phoning Dr. Robert Atkins, The Atkins Center for Complementary Medicine, New York City, NY, 1-201-285-4678 or the American College for Advancement in Medicine, 1-800-532-3688.

Following is a list of the vitamin supplements recommended by Dr. Anderson (in addition to 30 minutes of treadmill walking at a difficulty level of 2.5 on Monday, Wednesday, and Friday), which lowered my cholesterol count from 289 to 190 in three months. Today, the count is 157.

One Phosphatidyl Choline 425 mg	AM & PM
One Niacin (B3) Timed Release 500 mg	AM & PM
One Guggulipid 50 mg	PM
One Cayenne Pepper 500 mg	AM
Five Tablets Oat Bran 1 gram each	AM
One EPA Fish Oil 1000 mg	AM

My diet consisted of primarily protein, low unsaturated fats, and a moderate consumption of complex carbohydrates. The aerobic activity was comparable to a two-mile walk, which I prefer to do outdoors when the weather is fair, indoors on a treadmill when it is not. I interrupted the pace with a one-minute sprint at a treadmill difficulty level of 6. Lately, I have been able to bump that level to 7.5. An added bonus of visceral fat loss was noticeable when I walked before breakfast, probably due to my use of stored fat for energy. If the brain finds no dietary sugar for energy, it borrows sugar from stored fat deposits, which probably developed from years of excessive ingestion of simple carbohydrates. Like many of you, I was a sugarholic and really loved bread.

Of all the conjecture I read concerning diet, only one theory was proposed by a medical doctor, who had been trained in cardiology, that had enormous success in reducing the weight of the morbidly obese, and whose diet has been embraced by all intelligent medical practitioners for the treatment of diabetes. Dr. Robert Atkins was a rebel, though, who had locked horns indefatigably with the powerful AMA for taking a hard stand against our use of table sugar. Atkins pointed to an ominous correlation between the introduction of refined sugar to this country and the sudden rise of atherosclerosis (the blocking and hardening or the arteries). Apparently, he had also discovered that the form of political lobby taken by the U.S. sugar industry was to grant a generous annual stipend to the support of the Harvard Medical School. One does not like to bite the hand that feeds it.

Atkins and a small army of other alternative-choice physicians hurled another volley at the AMA by revealing a chemical drip procedure (EDTA) which can sweep the arterial walls clean of plaque. The AMA refuses to sanction this proven effective chelation procedure because it threatens to bankrupt the billion-dollar bypass industry. At this moment in time, over 500,000 American citizens are scheduled for heart bypass surgery. The operation and follow-up will cost them about $44,200 each. Chelation therapy has been proven to clear clogged arteries at a cost of $3,000 with no overnight hospitalization. The AMA ruthlessly branded Atkins and his followers with the steaming iron of "quackery," which, in turn, was largely responsible for the rebellion of avant-garde physicians and the birth of alternative or complementary medicine.

Atkins' preference for the high protein, low carbohydrate diet was not new. Ironically, he claims to have read about it in the hallowed *Journal of American Medicine*, adopting it to cure his own excessively fat condition. And surely he was familiar, as most nutritionally inquisitive readers were, with Dr. Irwin Stillman's 1967 *Quick Weight Loss Diet.* Stillman conquered his own obesity by lowering his carbohydrate consumption and drinking gallons of water. A decade later in 1977, Dr. Herman Tarnower corroborated with his low carbohydrate Scarsdale diet, implementing it to cure his own patients of arterial and heart disease.

Perhaps all of these gentlemen owe their success to an 1862 publication by William Banting, a British mortician, which was titled, *Letter on Corpulence.* With the Industrial Revolution creating affluent corporate giants in the Victorian period and into the early years of the 20th century, the portly businessman wore his corpulence like a badge of success. Banting's over-consumption of sugars and starches had ballooned his stomach so much he had to descend staircases backwards. Desperate, morbidly obese, he experimented with a high protein diet, eliminating starches and sweets, and lost over 50 pounds in just one year. Grinding the meat he ate to spread out consumption of it throughout the day led to the development of Salisbury steak, popular during the Victorian era; today, we call them hamburgers.

But the eradication of doubt about the efficacy of the high protein, low carbohydrate diet surely was pronounced by two courageous explorers of the Arctic in 1929, when they returned to report the absence of any carbohydrates in the winter diet of the Eskimo. Moreover, those natives were physically fit, strong, and without cardiovascular disease. Could their diet have been responsible for their unclogged arteries? To test this theory, Karsten Anderson and Vilhjalmur Stefanson, two Spartan adventurers, were monitored by physicians at New York's Bellevue Hospital for an entire year, during which time they ate nothing but a diet comprised of 25% protein and 75% fat. Results of their experiment showed no signs of cardiovascular malfunction, no rise in cholesterol or triglycerides, and both men had lost weight.

It is well known that the ingestion of sugar (or starch which is converted to sugar) excites the pancreas to churn out insulin, the primary metabolic hormone. Each of us has a specific tolerance for the ingestion of carbohydrates; too much, and the pancreas will deliver an excessive amount of insulin, which, in turn, attacks the sugar in our blood, leading to low blood sugar or hypoglycemia. We usually counter the resultant fatigue with the ingestion of more sugar. The overproduction of insulin elevates blood pressure, raises the triglyceride count, and produces low-density lipoproteins which, in turn, convert cholesterol to sticky plaque deposits on the walls of the arteries. Diabetes and obesity wait in the wings.

Despite the inaccurate reports you may have read about the diet theories of Dr. Atkins and his followers, at no time have we advocated a zero carbohydrate diet. We do encourage you to determine your own specific tolerance for carbohydrates and recommend that you do not exceed that level. You will soon learn how to determine your particular need for these macro nutrients.

Many of you live in some of the poorest states of the nation and simply cannot afford to eat a lot of protein. Your staple diet is high in carbohydrates. Women are noted for baking sugar-laden pies. Potatoes and spaghetti are frequent visitors to your plates, as well as corn, a high carbohydrate vegetable, and sterile white bread. Sweet apple cider often quenches your thirst, and maple syrup is sure to flow over your high stacks of pancakes. Even the occasional glass of orange juice fed to your children for vitamin C carries a whopping 27 grams of carbohydrates. Most of the food you are eating did not even exist 10,000 years ago. Industrial processing and public nutritional ignorance have changed the typical American silhouette. Many low-income women are obese, and their daughters are doomed to repeat the same ample silhouette because of their sugar and starch diet and lack of exercise. Diabetes is rampant in such areas, along with obesity and high blood pressure. Curiously, most of the husbands and sons in poor communities are lean. They do not all live long, though, and it has been our observation that many of them age rapidly. Close investigation has revealed that rural men work harder and longer than do men from the more cosmopolitan communities. The nature of their work, farming and construction, is physically demanding, and in the Northern states their six months of brutal winter is tortuous. Surely, they must be eating the same diets as their wives, yet most of the men appear to be lean. The obvious deduction is that the men are away from the kitchen most of the day. Their food is what fits in their lunch box, probably beef jerky. Most of these men have jobs that require strength and constant effort: anaerobic and aerobic activities. Both types of physical effort burn sugar, and when those supplies are depleted, these men become fat-burning engines. Small wonder they are lean. Excessive exercise with little rest invites muscle catabolism and destructive free radicals, though, and poor people cannot afford protective antioxidant supplements. These conditions are probably what age them rapidly.

We have explained how the ketogenic diet, most often referred to today as the "Atkins Diet," converts sugar-burning engines to fat-burning machines, fat being a far more efficient fuel as it is not burned as rapidly as sugar (carbohydrates of the "simple" variety). You probably will consume enough fat from the daily protein sources that you eat, and since we have identified saturated fat as a dangerous free radical magnet, we never advise ingestion of it as a food source in industrial, free radical proliferant communities. Rather, we prefer to restrict fat ingestion to fish oils, flax and olive oils, lecithin (in its concentrated high-potency form called phosphatidyl choline), evening primrose oil, and safflower, with an occasional shot of MCT (medium chain triglycerides) oil for energy. Other fats that I included during my twelve-month rejuvenation program are occasional nuts and avocado. It is the saturated fats that we try to avoid (fats that solidify at room temperature).

Protein is the principle dietary focus of the professional body-building community, with the muscular champions ingesting 2 to 3 grams of protein per pound of their massive body weight. The high-intensity pace that these men program in the gym rips their muscles with stress. The torn fibers rejuvenate through the process of protein synthesis, which also feeds previously dormant fibers to protect against new physical challenges; this is the basic science of muscle growth. To ingest such a vast amount of protein from solid foods alone would require an enormous appetite plus a huge stomach reservoir. The girth of power lifters' stomachs could be a result of such food volume distention. Since symmetry is more important to the professional body builder (and to the authors) than the astounding feats of strength that lure power lifters, wise body builders limit their food quantity by spreading consumption over six small-volume meals, rather than three large ones, and supplement their food protein with powdered protein supplements that are digested quickly; of these, the most rapidly assimilated form is comprised of hydrolyzed or pre-digested whey peptides. Whey peptides are short proteins composed of two or three different amino acids. The digestive system appears to absorb peptides more rapidly than whole proteins or singular amino acids. Therefore, muscle development, i.e., protein synthesis, can be accelerated with whey supplementation far more efficiently than from food protein, lessening the volume of the stomach cavity. It is precisely from such practice as limiting food quantity, albeit high in protein content, and increasing ingestion of ionized whey protein powders that Frank was able to diminish the diameter of his stomach, eliminate his visceral fat, and rediscover his abdominal wall of muscle. While he is still striving for "deeper cuts," the transition Frank made in six months is extraordinary.

Whey protein isolate is preferred to the whey protein concentrate, as the former will most assuredly provide 80% to 90% protein, while the concentrate variety usually includes high fat and/or high carbohydrates and lactose, rendering it lower in biological value. The isolate variety also provides more low molecular weight micro fractions, like IGF-I and II, glutathione, and bovine serum albumin, which can stimulate Growth Hormone activity and provide immune enhancement with vital antioxidants.

There are many whey protein products on the health food store shelves, and it would be indiscreet for us to plug any particular one. Following are some shopping parameters we would want you to consider if we were your personal trainers.

- Compare the quantity of one serving as it relates to a particular gram count of powder. One product might advertise that it contains 45 grams of protein per serving, while another might only claim 17 grams. But, if the first product calls one serving 72 grams and the second calls one serving 30 grams, the quantity of protein is close to being the same. Therefore, choose the product that offers the lower gram per serving, the lower price, or the one that includes glutamine and taurine, important for protein synthesis.
- Look for a low sodium count, certainly no higher than 350 mg per serving. The potassium count should be much greater.
- Choose a product, if you are training for lean muscle and low body fat, that has a low carbohydrate count; no more than 24 grams, preferably under 20 grams per serving. Ketogenic dieters can find protein powders that include less than 5 grams of carbohydrate per serving. Use only

water as the diluent and be sure to drink 10 added glasses of water per day. If you are ectomorphic and want to gain weight, supplementing with a high carbohydrate/protein powder will pack the pounds on fast, especially if you dilute the powder with milk. But it will not be all muscle. And if you are not training at high intensity, a large percentage of your subsequent weight gain will be fat.

- Alternate protein drinks that include glutamine with those that include creatine; powders that include both establish competition between each other for optimum digestibility. While creatine enhances strength and energy, volumizing muscle cells with water retention outside the cell wall, glutamine supplementation will help those cells maintain maximum volumization by preserving your muscles' most abundant amino acids within the cell. Glutamine and its synergist, taurine, keep the muscles in positive nitrogen balance (without which there can be no growth). When glutamine and taurine levels drop, protein can catabolize. These two important amino acids inhibit that process; their interference is called antiproteolysis. Catabolism of muscle is a natural result of chronic stress from intense training, if this stress is not nourished with protein, but ingested protein can catabolize if it is not protected with glutamine and taurine supplementation (Rowbottom, et al., 1996). Ten grams of glutamine per day promoted significant gains in Frank's strength and energy within one month. This gain may be attributed to the effect of glutamine upon gluconeogenesis (the creation of glucose from other sources). Glutamine becomes glutamate, which becomes alanine, which the liver converts to glucose, the energy source of muscle.
- Select a product that includes ionized, hydrolyzed or pre-digested whey. Might as well find one that tastes good, too!

The macro nutrient, protein, develops and maintains muscle and bone. High ingestion (one gram per pound of body weight is optimum, if you exercise) will boost your metabolic rate if spread over six meals. Unlike sugar and fat, protein cannot disrupt your blood sugar levels; it is thus a more lasting source of energy. A late conjecture suggests that combining whey protein with one from a casein source may protect against stress-related catabolism. The whey provides fast absorption for instant anabolic development, while the casein variety is more slowly digested, offering continuous resistance to the harmful effects of high-intensity muscle stress triggered by the release of the hormone cortisol. Like testosterone, cortisol is a steroid hormone derived from cholesterol and is produced by the adrenal glands in response to mental or physical stress.

Cortisol is classified as a glucocorticoid, since it breaks down protein (amino acids) and fatty acids into minute molecules to produce glucose, your body's primary source of energy. The problem is that the glucose sucks these vital acids directly from your muscles. That depletion, disintegrating muscle fiber, is the definition of muscle catabolism. High-intensity exercise (weight-resistance movements) partially protects against this phenomenon as it weakens the binding of cortisol to muscle cells, which volumize during such stress and increase the protective hormone testosterone. Other forms of exercise do not protect the muscle cells from cortisol, which accounts for the emaciated state of marathon runners and for the atrophy of a muscle that is bound in a cast to cure a bone injury. Cortisol, triggered by the stress of injury, devours lethargic muscle insatiably.

The primary reason professional body builders take steroids is that they occupy the same cell sites as cortisol, shutting out the muscle depleting stress hormone. Testosterone is the most powerful of these steroids, as it is highly anabolic. While excesses or abuse of steroids can be harmful to young athletes, older male readers may have a legitimate need for testosterone supplementation, as the levels of this male-specific hormone begin to decline after the age of 25, taking a drastic nose dive among the physically inactive through their senior years. You probably know some men of retirement age whose muscles are flaccid. Their voices become elevated, facial hair disappears, and their general countenance becomes more feminine, all opposite symptoms to those of a woman at menopause. Frank's rejuvenation as he enters his 68th year includes new muscle growth and a tripled strength level largely due to testosterone and growth hormone supplementation (his free testosterone and IGF-1 levels were pitifully low), a quadrupling of his protein intake (and elimination of high glycemic simple sugars) and, of course, four or five one-hour sessions in the gym every week pushing phenomenal poundages.

The only risk in replenishing naturally diminishing testosterone hormones of a male patient is potential hypertrophy of the prostate. Indeed, Frank's prostate did grow a few points several months after he started hormone replacement therapy. To stop this annoying process, Dr. Anderson advised him to increase his consumption of the herbs Saw Palmetto and Pygeum, replace injections of testosterone cypionate with a milder dose of testosterone cream, and add the power-stimulating 19-Norandrostenediol to his supplement schedule. Sure enough, Frank's PSA (prostrate specific antigen, a measure of prostate size) number dropped dramatically, as his strength increased. The 21st century will welcome a pharmaceutical procedure to shrink the prostate. Until then, men have a choice—protect and enhance your masculinity and strength with testosterone supplementation, but expect your prostate to grow along with your muscle, or become a woman in an old man's body. Frank opted for the former choice, when Dr. Anderson explained the dilemma. It should be mentioned that a slight enlargement of the strangling prostate is not a pre-cancerous development. Cancer also causes hypertrophy of the prostate, but enlargement is natural in all men of retirement age and hypertrophy is not necessarily carcinogenic. Since prostate enlargement seems to be a natural development of the aging process, protective herbs like Saw Palmetto should be on the daily supplemental list of every senior male; they lowered Frank's PSA level 5 points, startling even Dr. Anderson. The herbs really work!

Included in that list should, of course, be a minimum of 400 mg phosphatidyl serine, a remarkable oil that can raise testosterone and simultaneously lower the catabolic hormone cortisol when combined with weight-resistance exercise (see Fahey and Pearl, "Hormonal Effects of Phosphatidyl Serine During Two Weeks of Intense Training", *Medicine and Science in Sports and Exercise*, 1998, abstract #201, and Monteleone, Beinant, and Tanzilo, et. al., "Effects of Phosphatidyl Serine on the Neuroendocrine Response to Physical Stress in Humans", *Neuroendocrinology*, 1990; 52, pp. 243-248). Phosphatidyl serine also seems to reduce muscle soreness during exercise, permitting body builders to push themselves beyond the pain barrier. As will be explained in *Chapter Three*, before a muscle can grow, it must be literally torn from stress; it is during the recuperation or resting phase between exercise encounters that muscle grows with greater strength, as dormant fibers are recruited to guard against future impending stress. An added bonus from phosphatidyl serine supplementation is mental enhancement, an improved concentration capacity, and short term memory sharpness. Tests by Crook, et al. (1991) have revealed improved scores from several neuropsychological examinations (see also Crook, Tinklenberg, Yesavage, et. al., 1991). The therapeutic dosage recommended for weight resistance exercisers is 400 mg upon awakening and another 400 mg before retiring. Phosphatidyl serine is expensive, but so are beer and hard liquor; it is a question of values.

These observations would lead one to believe that obesity can be avoided by a regimen of vigorous physical activity, by food volume depletion and carbohydrate reduction, and that antioxidant supplementation is necessary to combat the production of free radicals that results from prolonged strenuous exercise. Is it possible that controlled physical exercise, with sufficient rest for recuperation, plus a natural diet rich in protein with micronutrient supplementation to combat free radicals might prolong life expectancy? Therein lies the theme of our book. We believe we have found the path to a longer life. The adjustments we have made in our lifestyles have resulted in the energy and physical fitness of men half our age, the mental alertness of college professors, and the peace and contentment that comes with a life free from stress. We can probably do little about our human life span (about 120 years) but we can prolong our life expectancy and certainly improve our journey to an advanced age.

Chapter One

Know Your Enemies

When Dr. Anderson started his practice 25 years ago, patients were concerned only about curing their existing medical problems. About 10 to 12 years ago, patients began to ask him for methods of prevention, how to protect themselves from diseases or illnesses through which they saw their loved ones or friends suffer, such as mental senility, cardiovascular disease, strokes, crippling arthritis, and cancer. Many of this new breed of inquisitive patients had read extensively about various medical conditions and alternative treatments and were looking for protective guidance in their quest for prolonged health and active longevity. While the quest has existed for years, we continue to search for the "fountain of youth," expecting medicine to help us live longer. Medical technology, through antibiotics, hormonal balance, microscopic laser surgery, and organ transplants, has extended our life expectancy to 72 years, still far from our nature-designed span.

As we approach the year 2000, science has demonstrated that we have the capacity to live to 120. The reason that we almost never achieve this full lifespan is that we have not known how to stop the aging process, which leaves us vulnerable to diseases that rob us of our strength and, ultimately, our full life expectancy. How does one intervene and interrupt this aging-disease-aging cycle? What constitutes aging? These questions were touched upon briefly in the *Foreword* and *Introduction* sections of this book.

Many aging characteristics occur when cells are permanently damaged by continual attacks from chemical particles called free radicals (also known as oxidants). Free radicals are aberrant molecules that are missing an electron and are desperately trying to snatch one from healthy whole molecules. These free radicals careen out of control through our bodies, attacking our cells relentlessly, turning their fats rancid, rusting their protein matrix, piercing their membranes and corrupting their genetic DNA code until the cells become dysfunctional, deteriorate, and die. Extensive research has been documented on this aspect of the aging process. Although aging is not caused by just one factor, Dr. Denham Harman of the University of Nebraska College of Medicine and

Dr. Bruce Ames from the University of California at Berkeley have collected data in support of the theory that aging is primarily caused by free radicals.

From where do free radicals come? The key element in the production of free radicals is oxygen. As your body performs its millions of chemical interactions in the presence of oxygen, free radicals are produced.

- Your body uses oxygen to breathe and produce energy; free radicals are an unavoidable passenger accompanying the process. When you have too many of them, they are harmful to you.
- The environment contains numerous substances that give us free radicals directly—or cause us to create them as a by-product of fighting off toxins. Examples: cigarette smoke, smog, carbon monoxide from automobiles, pesticides, and toxic wastes.
- Each time your body defends itself against a free radical, a new free radical is produced, unleashing a chain reaction that can severely damage or destroy your tissues, leading to the death or mutation of cells.

If not checked, free radicals will injure or destroy everything they touch. Free radicals can literally devastate your immune system, severely crippling your body's defenses against many degenerative diseases and the ravaging effects of aging. Other studies (1959) found that free radicals were directly implicated in such diseases as cancer, atherosclerosis, hypertension, Alzheimer's disease, arthritis, late-onset diabetes, and Parkinson's disease. It's frightening to think how powerful these free radicals are—and how far-reaching their effects are in our bodies.

This free radical theory was not widely accepted until evidence began to mount. In 1992, researchers at the University of Kentucky Medical Center made a breakthrough—the first direct evidence of free radicals in the body. These researchers showed that free radical attacks on proteins damaged physiological function in gerbils. In their experiments, they found that the level of oxidized protein in the brain increased as their lab gerbils aged, resulting in memory impairment. Researchers gave these older gerbils a compound that reduces oxidization. After treatment, the senior gerbils were restored to more youthful brain functions, and were able to wind through a maze at about the same rate as the younger gerbils. Thus, we have solid proof evidence of the existence and the effect of free radicals—and of the resultant debilitating conditions being reversible with the administration of antioxidant compounds. This revelation may be one of the most important of the 20th century.

Importance of Antioxidants

Since oxidation is the problem, the solution is obviously an "antioxidant." Your body has natural built-in antioxidant defenses composed of enzymes, vitamins A, C, E, beta-carotene, and trace minerals such as selenium and zinc; each of these plays a different, important role in your health. Beta-carotene, for instance (which converts to vitamin A), prevents the creation of free radicals in the first place. Vitamin C fortifies your body against harmful reactions to free radicals occurring inside the cells. Vitamin E and selenium combine to prevent further cell damage. Antioxidants are three times more effective as protectors:

1. **Antioxidants prevent free radical production** that results from oxidation. You can observe the protective power of antioxidants by doing a little kitchen science. Crush a 500 mg tablet of vitamin C, or use one teaspoonful of the crystalline form. Next, cut an apple or pear in half and immediately spread a thin coat of the powdered vitamin C on the cut side of one half. Let both sit side by side and examine them after 15 minutes or so. The half "protected" by vitamin C will remain white and fresh, while the "unprotected" half will turn light brown, then dark brown as it reacts to the assault of oxygen. The same thing happens inside your body, not only to your food, but to your organs, as oxygen and the resulting free radicals do their deadly work within.
2. **Antioxidants put out the fire**. Antioxidants interrupt the damaging chain reaction started by free radicals. This interruption is particularly important when the free radicals attack the lipid (fat) layer of your cell membranes. As Frank mentioned, fat is a free radical magnet. Since lipid molecules are so concentrated in the membrane, the entire cell would be destroyed were it not for antioxidants, particularly vitamin E. Like water extinguishing flame, antioxidants put out the fire.
3. **Antioxidants scavenge free radical particles and neutralize them** before they have a chance to regenerate and do damage. A major antioxidant, beta-carotene, is particularly effective in neutralizing singlet oxygen, a reactive particle capable of generating and being transformed into more toxic-free radicals. Beta-carotene acts like a bullet-proof vest that can stop the single oxygen projectile.

Other factors known to be responsible for accelerating the aging process include:

alcohol	stress	nutritional deficiencies
smoking	radiation	ischemia
infection	electromagnetic exposure	lack of exercise
chronic disease	depression	hormone imbalance

Measurable changes that occur in our bodies as we age include the following:

These levels decline:	These levels increase:
Thymus gland	Breakdown of collagen
Estrogen/Progesterone	Ischemia
Testosterone	Autoantibodies
DHEA	Cortisol
Thyroid	Percentage of body fat
Melatonin	
ATP* production	
Glucose utilization and tolerance	
Human Growth Hormone	

*Adenosine Triphosphate—various compounds involved in the storage and transfer of energy in cells and muscles.

Stages of Aging

The stages of aging are based upon:

1. **Genetic Inherited Susceptibilities**. At present, we are unable to create genetic changes, but medical technology promises us in the not-too-distant future to be able to alter or transform our DNA genetic code. Obviously, this technique will have a major impact on how we treat or prevent diseases to enhance our mental and physical longevity. One major obstacle to this development is the liberal lobby of Moral Activists who condemn genetic experimentation.
2. **Cumulative Oxidative Damage by Free Radicals (Oxidants)**. We have learned how to neutralize or control free radicals by changing our lifestyle choices and behavior, as well as increasing our antioxidant levels through appropriate diet, vitamins, and exercise.
3. **Decline of Metabolic and Hormone Functioning**. In the last five years we have become much more knowledgeable of how our bodies work. We have learned the importance of hormone replacement and balancing and how these life-giving messengers, which are naturally and constantly standing guard in our bodies, promise active health and longevity if they are replenished. We predict that Hormone Replacement Therapy will become as commonplace as Tylenol in the 21stcentury. Celebrities have already discovered this Fountain of Youth. Read on. You may want to soon join them.

The next logical question one might ask, then, is why, with our new knowledge and technology we cannot live forever. In the natural universal order of things, as we get older, two critical things happen biologically to hasten aging and eventually cause death:

1. The rate of increase of cell-damaging free radical reactions accelerates drastically, especially in industrial communities and in smoke-clouded cities like Paris, where art museums are the only refuge for non-smokers.
2. Our inborn abilities to defuse and repair the damage from these free radicals, our detoxification systems, decline as we age. Therefore, the

older we get, the more damage accumulates in our cells, and the more the aging process accelerates.

The clock of life never stops ticking. In medicine, time is critical. Cells that have died in our vital organs cannot be replaced. The junk you eat today, your personal debilitating habits, like smoking, consumption of excessive alcohol, or lack of exercise can damage your life forever. Look at their elimination as a biochemical make-over or as internal surgery. It is not too late. The physical composition of the body can be changed by biochemical manipulation, through appropriate diet, nutritional supplements, lifestyle choices like the avoidance of smoking and drinking, and by following an exercise program, such as we have designed for you in a later chapter.

Smoking

It is hard to discuss longevity and aging without talking about smoking, for as you probably know, there are many hazards directly resulting from this foolish practice. Statistics from the National Center for Health:

- Each cigarette steals away 8 minutes of life.
- A pack a day equates to losing a month of life each year; 2 packs means 12 to 16 years off life expectancy for lifetime smokers.
- Just one cigarette can increase the heart rate 20 to 25 beats per minute and raise blood pressure significantly.
- Smoking one pack a day depletes more vitamin C (500 mg) than most people ingest in a day.
- Cigarettes raise carbon monoxide levels in the blood, which competes with oxygen so thoroughly that it takes the circulatory system 6 hours to return to normal after just one cigarette. Compound this result with the air contaminated by automobile exhaust and you will understand why city people age and die more rapidly than country farmers.
- Smoking is so immunosuppressive that it takes three months to reverse its damage to the immune system, when a smoker kicks the habit.

Second-hand Smoke

Secondary cigarette smoke inhaled by non-smokers can also pose health hazards.

- Secondary smoke has been linked to 20% of all lung cancers—this percentage equates to 3,000 lung cancer deaths each year among non-smokers, including children raised in the homes of smokers.
- Secondary smoke also causes 150,000 to 300,000 cases of respiratory illness, such as bronchitis, pneumonia, and asthma.
- Secondary smoke in a home that includes babies and children is a flagrant form of child abuse. Smokers should ask themselves: Am I killing my family?

Obesity

Obesity is thc second leading cause of preventable death in the United States, exceeded only by cigarette smoking. Obesity affects 58 million people in our nation and its prevalence is increasing. Obesity is a major determinant of premature mortality and must be addressed if one wishes to have active health and longevity.

Obesity is a major risk factor for cardiovascular disease, stroke, diabetes mellitus, and some cancers, contributing to 300,000 deaths annually in the United States. We have learned that obesity results from a complex interaction of genetic, behavioral, and environmental factors.

Because human nature is selfish, hedonistic, and often lethargic, exercise, diet and behavioral modification alone often are not sufficient to maintain long-term weight loss. Reluctant to admit to contempt, overweight patients prefer to acknowledge their condition as an illness. This false concept has led some doctors to oblige and identify obesity as a chronic disease, requiring medical intervention. In most cases, however, elimination of sugar and saturated fat will reduce body weight, so the real problem is truly one of contempt and self-gratification. Excess sugar ingestion will lead to fat storage in adipose tissue and triglycerides. Saturated fat also begets body fat. THE SATURATED FAT AND PROCESSED SUGAR THAT YOU ATE IS THE FAT THAT YOU CURRENTLY WEAR. Exercise alone will not reduce body fat. We just have to learn how to eat sensibly.

Primitive man lived on protein and fat, much like the Eskimo of the Tundra has for centuries. You cannot plant corn on ice. Bread is man's invention, not nature's. All flour products are inventions of man (or woman). All processed foods are man's contribution to the food chain. Before farming, man of the Ice Age stood tall on thick bones that suggest thick musculature. Later prehistoric remains are smaller, grotesquely revealing a history of osteoporosis and arthritis. The more meals that the woman prepared in the cave, the less motivation did her mate have to hunt for protein sources. As the chase became less frequent, his body began to waste with atrophy. In the name of Industrial Civilization, man began to process foods, adding chemicals to prevent spoilage. He fattened his farm animals with steroids and stuffed the mouths of his children with sugar to elicit their love and dependence. Is it any wonder that we contract diseases? We truly are what we eat. Your children are what you feed them.

Sugar and fat are your primary enemies. Most citizens are protein-deficient, sugar-burning machines. Protein will give you strength and good fats, like fish oils, will provide far more efficient energy than sugar. Following are some ways to skim the saturated fat and simple sugars from your daily diet:

Food item:	**Switch from:**	**To a better choice:**	**But aim for:**
Dairy	whole milk	2% milk	No milk at all; if you are an adult, you do not need it.
	processed cheese	reduced fat or hard cheese	Fat-free cheese; occasional hard cheese.
	ice cream	ice milk, frozen yogurt	Low-fat ice cream or fat-free frozen yogurt (plain).
	sour cream	reduced fat sour cream	Low-fat sour cream or no sour cream;
	yogurt	low-fat yogurt	plain yogurt (add your own fruit).
Eggs* For cholesterol-emics only! (Cooked whole eggs in moderation are fine for healthy individuals.)	2 whole eggs	1 whole egg and I egg white	egg substitute, egg whites (package in dairy case)
Fats	butter	less butter	no butter
	mayonnaise	reduced fat mayo	fat-free mayo
	margarine	canola oil	olive oil or flaxseed oil

Desserts & Snacks	creamy dips corn/potato chips cookies sugar candies	low-fat yogurt-based dip light popcorn reduced-fat cookies fruit	salsa pretzels, hot-air popcorn (both in moderation) graham crackers, fig bars, ginger snaps, fat-free cookies, all in low quantity low-carb fruit
Grains	croissant, donut	bagel English muffin	whole grain toast, multi-grain crackers
Fruit	grapes pears pineapple	bananas nectarines grapefruit, apples	Cantaloupe plums strawberries
Meat	bacon, sausage pastrami bologna, salami fatty pork	corned beef lean ham, Canadian bacon 98% fat-free meat filet mignon fat-free bologna	low-fat turkey-bacon and sausage any kind of fish, seafood, or fowl

*Frank lowered his cholesterol over 100 points in 3 months while ingesting an average of one dozen eggs per week.

Get Your Share of Antioxidant Foods

You can get many anti-aging nutrients you need from a variety of foods:

Beta-Carotene/Vitamin A
Carrots, winter squash
Broccoli, cauliflower, cabbage
Romaine lettuce, kale
Apricots, nectarines, peaches
Swiss chard, collard
Crab, whitefish
Bran flakes
Tomatoes

Vitamin E
Leafy greens
100% whole wheat bread
Wheat germ
Almonds, hazelnuts
Vegetable oil
Cucumbers
Brown rice
Asparagus
Green peas

Zinc
Oysters
Wheat germ
Ground mustard
Beans, lentils
Brewer's yeast
Oats, oatmeal
Pumpkin seeds, sunflower seeds
Mushrooms
Popcorn
Non-fat, dry milk

Vitamin C
Cantaloupe
Broccoli, Brussels sprouts
Cabbage, cauliflower
Peppers
Fruit juices
Potato baked in skin
Strawberries, boysenberries
Black currants
Wheat flakes
Asparagus

Selenium
Chicken breast or turkey
Brown or white rice
Salmon, tuna
Shrimp, oysters
Whole wheat, bran
Garlic, onions
Vinegar, molasses
Cottage cheese
Mushrooms

Caution: Yellow vegetables like corn are high in carb content. Juices carry twice the carbohydrate as their whole fruit counterparts. Cantaloupe, plums and strawberries are the lowest in carbs; grapes and pears the highest.

Nutritional Supplements to Fight Free Radicals

In addition to the right foods, we believe you should also take antioxidant nutritional supplements. It is not enough to take the Food and Drug Administration's (FDA) recommended daily allowance (RDA). Their guidelines are to barely stay alive.

The government's RDAs are the minimum requirements for marginally functional people and do not take into account that over half the population is already "sick" with heart disease, osteoporosis, arthritis, or some other degenerative disease. Marginally functional people also differ markedly in their individual profiles. Nor did the designers of RDAs consider that many Americans breathe dirty air, drink polluted water, and eat chemically treated food—all potent sources of free radicals that demand supplemental protection.

If you care about your health and longevity (and who doesn't!), you will want to take enough antioxidants to really rid your body of free radicals—and not just enough to satisfy the government's RDA. Dr. Anderson recommends the following daily minimum doses to his patients:

Vitamin C:	3,000 mg spread throughout the day
Beta-Carotene:	15,000 iu
Vitamin E:	400 iu
Selenium:	200-400 mcg
Zinc:	30 mg

Frank has followed a similar schedule for over 25 years. He spreads the vitamin C <u>throughout</u> the day (during meals), as it is quickly absorbed and excreted by your body. Ester-C is the most potent variety. We also recommend a high-potency multi-vitamin/mineral supplement, and a potent B-complex tablet daily (100 mg minimum).

There are three key things to remember for good antioxidant defense against aging. I hope you will take these suggestions seriously because we are not just talking here about winning a football game—we're talking about your health and life.

Key#1: Eat a low-fat diet. While fat may have been eaten by primitive man, he had no outside pollution with which to contend. Pollution breeds aggressive free radicals. Saturated fat is a magnet for free radicals, so a low-fat diet can reduce your intake of free radicals. Atherosclerosis, cancer, arthritis, Parkinson's disease, and even cataracts, are also associated with increased intake of saturated fat. It is likely that the fat itself is not at fault, but rather that it attracts free radicals. Not all fats are bad for you. Good fats include Omega-3 and Omega-6 fatty acids, linoleic and linolenic acids, oils like flax, EPA (eicosapentanoic acid), DHA (docosahexaoic acid), and safflower; these will provide energy for fat burning engines and should be a part of your stable diet.

Key #2: Do not smoke, and avoid inhaling smoke from someone else's cigarette. Tell your smoking friends and relatives that they are always welcome in your home, but that their cigarettes are not. If they truly love you, they will comply. If you truly love them, encourage them to quit. The toxins in cigarette smoke can be a deadly source of free radicals in your body You and your teenager are consuming them every time you visit a bar or attend a rock concert. The axiom is: Be cool, be dead.

Key #3: Get on a program of regular physical activity. Anaerobic training with weight resistance will speed up your metabolism (even while resting). Resulting thermogenesis (body cells creating heat energy) will enable your body to run more efficiently in every way. You will experience stronger resistance to free radicals and counteract the primary characteristics of aging. There is no better form of exercise than training with weights, but consider blending your workouts with cross-training that includes pleasurable sports and outdoor activity. Muscle is a vital defense against the aging process. Inactivity results in atrophy of muscle and physical deterioration. What you do not use, you will most certainly lose. Remember, you are the sculptor of your own countenance.

Chapter Two

Defenses Against Biological Debilitation

"Old age must be resisted and its deficiencies restored."

Cicero, Marcus
Roman philosopher (106-43 B.C.)

Hormonal Therapy

Dr. Anderson's 25 years as a practicing physician has taught him that nothing which happens in our body occurs as an isolated event. One change leads to a cascade of events that can eventually be felt in every cell of every organ throughout our entire body; this is precisely what happens when the aging clock runs down and the levels of our body's hormones decline. We experience profound changes that affect every aspect of our physical and mental well-being. These changes are reflective not only in our behavior, but also in our outlook on life itself. We lose what Dr. Anderson refers to as the "eye of the tiger." We lose the joie de vivre, in other words, our psychic energy. We lose the mental vitality that keeps us motivated and being part of the exciting world in which we live. We lose our desire to learn and try new things. We become set in our ways. I believe it is the loss of this psychic energy which is responsible for the fear of trying something new. As we age, we feel overwhelmed by new experiences and we respond by trying to avoid them. Life becomes monotonous; it should not and need not be this way. Let us introduce you to the super hormones and the miraculous changes that these can effect.

What are hormones? As most people know, our bodies are run by hormones which are responsible for our sexuality. Hormones give us our body shape, determine our voice—whether it is a high or a low pitch, help regulate our sleep, our mental status, our moods, our memory, our libido and much more. Hormones, however, are also known to impact many of the human aging parameters, the discoveries that have become so exciting in just the last few years. We want to explore these discoveries in depth and look at the great potential they have for all of us as we enter the 21st century.

When we talk about hormones, we are not promoting testosterone magnifying steroids, harmful, unnatural drugs foolishly fed into the vascular system of professional bodybuilders from the anabolic steroid era (Anadrol, Dianabol or Deca-Durabolin, etc.). These steroids are currently rated illegal by the FDA, providing a history of serious side effects. While they did build bodies of gargantuan proportions, these silhouettes can hardly be referred to as natural. There are natural hormones that have regulated everyone's body from birth, which, as we age, go through numerous reductive changes. We have the ability to monitor these hormones and to supplement them, giving ourselves a regenerative, stronger life with active health and longevity. The hormones that we will consider in this book are the thyroid hormone, melatonin (released into the blood by the pineal gland in the brain), dehydroepiandrosterone (DHEA, produced by the pituitary gland of the brain) pregnenolone, estrogen, progesterone, testosterone and its precursors. We will also emphasize the importance of the Human Growth Hormone (HGH), about which so much research has been done within the last few years.

Thyroid

One of the most prevalent basic ailments and one of the least diagnosed conditions that contribute to horrendous medical costs and, for many people, gradual deterioration, is a condition of low thyroid function, also known as hypothyroidism. There are more than 64 symptoms of low thyroid function, the most prevalent of which are some of today's most common disorders, such as fatigue and depression. Hypothyroidism is a widespread illness that basically can sap you of physical vigor, reduce your sexual vitality, steal your ability to think, to remember, and can undermine your total emotional life. Although we encourage you to take more responsibility for your health, seeking wellness from thyroid supplementation should be done in cooperation with a complementary physician, of course. More physicians are becoming aware of the benefits that can result from preventive methods, among them nutrition and hormone supplementation. Look for a physician who is aware of the various ways of evaluating and stimulating the thyroid.

We have found that the typical traditional laboratory testing of the thyroid, with its T3, T4 and TSH levels indicated in a patient's blood, is not the only way to evaluate the performance of a thyroid. For many years Dr. Broda Barnes did a phenomenal amount of research on the subject. A medical doctor, as well as a Ph.D., Barnes developed what we refer to as the Barnes basal temperature test, which involves taking your body temperature first thing in the morning after a good night's sleep, tucking the thermometer snugly in your arm pit for ten minutes as you lie there. If your thyroid function is normal, your temperature should be in the range from 97.8 to 98.2 degrees Fahrenheit, if lower, you may be hypothyroid. This condition exists because your thyroid gland is under-functioning, and a lot of your physical problems and related feelings could be caused, or at least be influenced, by an underactive thyroid. This underarm test, even though it sounds extremely simple, has been painstakingly checked for accuracy against basal metabolism results of thousands of persons in the early 1940s. The writers have read many papers on the subject published in numerous prestigious medical journals, all testifying to its efficacy.

As an alternative physician, Dr. Anderson has learned that, even though the temperature test's accuracy has been abundantly demonstrated, one should not rely exclusively upon its results. He verifies these results by looking for classical symptoms of an underactive hypothyroid, based on the patient's thorough medical history, with careful correlation and interpretation of the data. All of our blood (approximately five quarts) circulates through the thyroid gland once every hour, bringing iodine, the material your thyroid needs to make hormones, as well as a hormone from the anterior pituitary gland called the thyroid stimulating hormone, which stimulates production from the thyroid gland. The thyroid also stores and discharges thyroid hormone in the blood stream for delivery to your cells where and when it is needed. Too little thyroid hormone, in the case of hypothyroidism, causes your motor to run sluggishly; the heartbeat slows, blood pressure drops, circulation becomes lazy, contributing to discomfort from cold, particularly in the hands and feet. Energy levels and endurance are low. Digestion slows down. Constipation becomes common. Headaches occur frequently. Hair can become lifeless, falling out more readily. Nails become brittle. Wounds heal slowly. Thinking becomes slower. Memory is undependable, and your sex urge becomes weak or dormant. The effects of hypothyroidism are felt in each and every one of our trillions of cells and every organ and tissue of our body.

One case history that comes to Dr. Anderson's mind was Andrew, a 13-year-old freshman from the Southern part of Vermont, who came to see him with a history of depression, lack of motivation, and persistent cold-like symptoms. He had seen numerous physicians, including a psychiatrist, and all his blood work was normal. He had been on numerous antibiotics and Prozac, all to no avail. Upon first seeing this young man, it was quite apparent that he was not your typical teenager. He was pale, over-dressed for the office temperature, attached to a box of tissues, and had a lethargic response during his interview. Dr. Anderson asked his mom to take the boy's basal body temperature for five mornings before Andrew got out of bed and to phone in the results. His temperatures were consistently between 95 and 96 degrees. At school, the nurse documented his body temperature, which was 97.8 on numerous occasions at mid-day. The doctor started Andrew on Armour Thyroid (¼ grain) and the results were phenomenal. The following is a letter from his mother who clearly describes the transformation of Andrew:

> Dear Dr. Anderson:
>
> Andrew is feeling and doing so much better than he has in years. He has not gotten sick with a staph infection or any chronic type of infection since he has started on thyroid treatment. The runny nose and "cold" that he had for 11 months has gone and has not returned. He no longer displays the nearly comatose level of exhaustion that kept him appearing depressed and disinterested in life. He is not always cold, and his temperature is not below normal all the time His concentration has improved, and he has only missed two days of school this year. His pupils are no longer dilated; his skin no longer gray and without any trace of color; his skin is not so dry anymore.
>
> Andrew was previously diagnosed by mainstream physicians as being "EBD" or emotionally/behaviorally disturbed. His exhaustion was perceived by them to be a type of conduct behavior disorder (avoidance), because he could not apply himself to his work, and some school personnel believed he was "playing games" to avoid working, using exhaustion as an excuse. I might add that his stomach aches have just about gone away, as well as have his stomach cramps, since his thyroid problem was diagnosed.
>
> He has tested academically in the superior, if not gifted, ranges in all areas, missing an accumulation of probably nearly one-third, if not more, of his education being absent from school. Because of his previously low performance, however, and inability to perform in school (again, seen by some as refusal), he has been labeled emotionally/behaviorally disturbed.
>
> Andrew has always been pleasant and cooperative, and his lethargy and lack of motivation combined with his high IQ has been a real mystery. Thank

> you for your help, Dr. Anderson. Andrew is a different person today because you took the time to look, listen and investigate. Before the thyroid diagnosis, he was without hope and too exhausted to get through a single day; his brain was foggy and he could not concentrate. Now his health and energy are being restored and he wants to succeed in life. (personal correspondence, 1998).

Conversely, too much thyroid hormone, a condition known as hyperthyroidism, makes the motor race, increasing the heartbeat, raising blood pressure and swelling blood volume. You flush from overheating, often to the level of a mild fever. You perspire profusely, are nervous and sleepless, and may even have episodes of diarrhea.

As one gets older, the condition of an underactive thyroid gland, again, hypothyroidism, is quite common, affecting one out of every four women over the age of 40 and one of every 10 men. This condition is of great significance. If we wish to go forward with active health and longevity, we must occasionally monitor our thyroid hormone, checking, as we awaken, our basal body temperature, and we must supplement ourselves, when needed, with thyroid hormone. Controversy, however, exists as to what type of thyroid hormone should be used—the synthetic, which can give you either T3 alone or a T4 in the form of either Synthroid or Cytomel. Most alternative physicians prefer to use desiccated thyroid. The company that has been supplying this for many years is Armour; their thyroid supplement is a combination ofT3 and T4. Dr. Anderson typically starts the patient on one-quarter grain of the Armour thyroid. After a couple of weeks, monitoring both the blood work as well as the clinical symptoms of the patient when they return, along with their basal body temperature, he determines whether or not he needs to increase the dosage.

In order to get the maximum benefit from your thyroid gland, either by itself or with supplementation, other vitamins that are very important for its efficiency are A, the B vitamins, specifically vitamin B_2, B_6 and B_{12}, and also vitamin C. That combination will enhance your own natural thyroid circulating hormone when taken with supplementation of the thyroid hormone from Armour. The primary benefit of supplemental thyroid for all of us is mainly that of energy production and also has been shown to help control cholesterol and triglyceride levels; it does have a strong impact on lowering them. Also, the supplement has a direct relationship with our libido. A close and sympathetic relationship exists between the thyroid and the sexual glands of men and women. Sexual function really is an expression of energy, and due to the fact that the thyroid is the governor of our uses of energy, we should not be too surprised by this association. In reality, sexual attractiveness is triggered by alertness, animation, fire and sparkle seen in someone of the opposite sex, all of which can be a result of the condition and state of our thyroid gland.

We have also learned that one of the benefits of thyroid supplementation is weight loss for people who are having difficulty losing weight. Many times these overweight persons will have a body fat status baseline. They reach a certain level or set point, and, regardless of what they do, using medication, practicing strict selection and food awareness, and even through consistent and persistent exercise, they are still not able to break below a certain stratosphere of weight. We have learned many times that supplemental thyroid can be of benefit in enhancing these people's weight loss programs. Too often, the level of the thyroid hormone is drawn and measured from blood drawn by a physician and found to be normal. The patient is then informed that their thyroid is normal. As Dr. Anderson has learned, and expressed earlier, this information is often a fallacy that he has proven many times by using the basal body temperature test, revealing that the patient's thyroid is underactive.

Dr. Anderson adds:

> In starting an ameliorative program, I begin patients on one-quarter grain of thyroid, then monitor them in a couple of weeks. They are advised to exercise, practice selective food awareness and seek nutritional counseling. Many times we have brought about a significant reduction in a patient's weight. The patient becomes motivated when initially seeing some pounds lost. This achievement seems to self-perpetuate, and really is quite beneficial in regulating a new, more desired body weight set point.
>
> The thyroid hormone also stimulates protein synthesis, which is necessary for the buildup of muscle from amino acids. Protein is necessary for replacing worn out cells and for the manufacture of enzymes, which moderate the speed at which many biochemical reactions take place within the cells. Thyroid hormone also potentiates the effect of other body hormones, such as adrenaline. It is necessary for the secretion of sex-activating hormones, such as the gonadotropins of the pituitary gland (those that cause testes and ovaries to act). Thyroid hormone is also, in large part, responsible for controlling the rate of absorption of nutrients in the gastrointestinal tract.

So, the importance of thyroid function to good health should not be underestimated. The thyroid gland is the largest endocrine gland in the human body, weighing less than one ounce, secreting less than a teaspoon of hormone substance a year, yet it controls the metabolic activity of all of our cells.

Cellular health, when you think about it, depends really upon three major factors: oxygen, nutrients, and the function of the thyroid hormones. Supplemental thyroid hormone counteracts oxidated metabolism, thereby increasing oxygen consumption within every cell.

We recommend that all patients, especially if you are approaching your fourth and fifth decade of life, have a screening for hypothyroidism. Included in the screening, not to be redundant, should be both blood work and basal body temperature screening. Find a complementary physician who will sit down and clearly listen to your symptoms. In any program where you wish to receive and achieve active health and longevity, you must have a normally working thyroid gland or proper thyroid supplementation, for thyroid hormone is a necessity for every cell, tissue and organ in our body.

Dehydroepiandrosterone (DHEA)

You probably recognize the name of this hormone because there is scarcely a health or fitness magazine, news article, radio or TV program that has not been talking about the controversial benefits of DHEA. To begin with, DHEA is produced by the pituitary gland of the brain, released by the adrenal cortex of our bodies, and it is the most abundant hormone in our body, a precursor to many of the sex hormones, testosterone, estrogen, and progesterone. We have realized that our levels of DHEA reach their highest point when we are in the prime of our life, which is approximately 18 to 25 years of age. During this period of time, the normal male produces approximately 31 mg of DHEA on a daily basis, and the normal female produces approximately 19 mg of DHEA. If doctors supplement their patients with DHEA, they should first be aware of what their daily production was during their prime. This awareness, along with blood tests or saliva tests that measure present levels, helps physicians to prescribe what dosage of supplementation is most efficacious.

Current research has shown that DHEA is of great value in preventing and treating cardiovascular diseases, elevated cholesterol, diabetes, osteoporosis, obesity, Alzheimer's disease, enhancement of our immune system, and perhaps most interestingly, DHEA is currently being investigated as an effective anti-aging hormone (Abbasi, et al., *Journal of the American Geriatric Society*, 1998). Touted by many as a wonder drug, DHEA must not be considered a magic bullet and should only be taken under medical supervision. Patients may have their blood or saliva levels measured to determine their specific need. DHEA, as we know, is a hormone, and hormones affect many things in the body. No one should start playing around with their hormonal balance without guidance from a complementary physician. Furthermore, as we mentioned, DHEA is a hormone precursor, meaning that it can turn into other hormones in the body. Like testosterone or estrogen, DHEA affects everyone differently. It can, for instance, if a dose is frequent and excessive, create a testosterone overload which can be damaging to a woman's health, creating unpleasant side effects like facial hair, acne, deepening of the voice, and changing of her female anatomy. Surplus testosterone augmented by DHEA supplementation can also increase the size of the prostate in men, so keep an eye open for your PSA count should you begin a DHEA and testosterone supplementation program. The herbs Saw Palmetto and Pygeum can decrease enlarged prostates. As we reported earlier, they lowered Frank's PSA five points; include them if you are a male close to 50.

Levels of DHEA production in the body vary accordingly to stress, fever, sudden lowering of blood sugar and disease states. DHEA levels are also lower among smokers than among nonsmokers and are especially lower among people who drink a great amount of alcohol. We have learned that birth control pills and other synthetic hormones also deplete our DHEA levels. DHEA has a long half-life of approximately 8 to 11 hours, due to its slow clearance in our body by the liver and kidneys, and therefore its adequate consumption is usually once a day. Dr. Anderson tries to mimic his patients bodies circadian rhythm, usually recommending DHEA supplementation in the evening. For some patients, however, DHEA is too much of a stimulant, and they should take DHEA either in the morning or afternoon hours.

The benefits of DHEA replacement are very similar to those resulting from Human Growth Hormone therapy. A great majority of hormone recipients reported a vast improvement in their mood and energy, but even more impressive was the effect of DHEA replacement on the subjects' Human Growth Hormone levels. Studies such as those by Dr. Omid Khorram, former University of California, San Diego Professor of Medicine, report that restoring DHEA levels to youthful levels in elderly men and women greatly increased their blood levels of insulin growth factor-1 (IGF-1) (Khorram, Vu and Yen, 1996). This protein, you may know, is a product of Human Growth Hormone secretions. The levels of IGF-I give a very accurate measure of the amount of HGH in the body. It can be assumed that DHEA can increase the levels of HGH, which may partly account for the all encompassing reported benefits of

DHEA treatment. The amount of increase is largely dependent upon your age. If you are into your late 50's or 60's, your ability to produce HGH is often depleted. If it is, no amount of DHEA supplementation will elevate your Human Growth Hormone secretions significantly, nor will it greatly increase your blood levels of IGF-1. So, HGH benefits are largely dependent upon what age you are when you start taking the product, and how you stand physically. This is one of the reasons why you should certainly have your blood or saliva levels checked for your personal need for DHEA level supplementation. You do not want to be taking extra DHEA if you are already at an adequate level. Superfluous supplements can actually impede your own body's production of DHEA. Obviously, it would be ludicrous to suppress something in your body that is already being produced by supplementing with something similar that you purchase at a store.

As we discussed earlier, DHEA supplementation also has been reported by many recipients to improve sexual function. DHEA has been considered a "mother hormone," since it is a precursor to the sex hormones and supplementation can raise the levels of testosterone, estrogen and progesterone to youthful amounts. By supplementing with DHEA and raising the levels of sex hormones, sexual function, including erection, lubrication and orgasm can all be improved. You may not need Viagra.

Another reported benefit from those who do take the DHEA supplementation has been weight reduction (Ciore, *Obesity Research*, 1995). This weight-reducing mechanism may operate through the increase of serotonin levels in the hypothalamus region of our brain, thereby increasing the release of Cholecystokinin, which is the satiation hormone that decreases one's desire for food by creating a feeling of fullness. When we talk about weight loss from DHEA supplementation, we are not talking about a great deal of poundage, but in Dr. Anderson's experience, many patients have lost somewhere in the range of five to perhaps eight pounds after a few months of supplementation. Some women have happily reported spot fat loss from their hips and thighs following DHEA supplementation. This loss can be related to its androgenic effect (*Muscle and Fitness*, 1996), challenging the dogma that spot reduction of fat is impossible. Better limit your daily dosage to no more than 25 mg, though, girls, or you may have to buy a shaving kit for your face.

DHEA also has a strong influence on the functioning of our brain, because there is more DHEA in the tissues of the brain than in any other tissues of the body. Optimum DHEA levels have improved memory and mental acuity.

These studies have been confirmed by various researchers using mice as their subjects, showing that supplemental DHEA activated the growth of interneuron connectors. The more of these connectors there are in the brain, the quicker the communication and the transfer of information between brain cells. Other studies have been done on humans who were suffering from depression and memory problems. After treating these persons with DHEA, it was noted that most of the depression had dramatically improved, as well as the collective and incidental memory. Because these are the first two types of memory to deteriorate in patients who suffer from Alzheimer's disease, DHEA could prove to be very helpful in treating or preventing this serious debilitating mental condition (Holsboer, et al., 1994).

This powerful hormone also, as we stated earlier, boosts our immune system by controlling the production of the stress hormones, adrenaline and cortisol. Stress hormones are released by the adrenal glands and raise the body's blood sugar, and increase our heart rate in order to prepare the body to cope with the fight or flee mechanism. Ideally, all of these hormones are used up in dealing with the stressor, usually in physical output. When the hormones are not used up, we internalize our stress and cannot act upon it physically. With an unhealthy buildup of stress hormones, the body's immune response becomes inhibited, and the T cells, which fight off infections, do not work as well as they should, thus allowing us to become more susceptible to illness. When a person comes down with something as simple as a common cold, if you look back at what took place in the few days prior to that event, you can often recall some excessive stress, whether it be long hours, some very stressful situations at work, or something stressful going on financially or emotionally in a person's life. Stress can be such a debilitating agent for so many of us, that in addition to looking at stress and treating it with the use of micronutrient or hormonal supplementation, we also have learned to recognize the extraordinary benefits of using spiritual meditation or prayer to help a stressed person relax.

For your use of DHEA, I must reiterate that it is our opinion that you have yourself monitored by a qualified physician. Have your blood or saliva level checked to see exactly where your status is. Then go about using appropriate supplementation, if it is indicated. For most females, the dosage is in the vicinity of approximately 10 mg on a daily basis, and for most men the range is usually between 10 and 25 mg. Physically active men and women may need much more. Some early signals that your supplementation may be too high would be that of acne, increased facial hair, increased frequency of headaches, and also some irritability, shortness of temper or change in mood. Dr. Anderson prescribed 25 mg for Frank after his first blood test indicated a dire need. Six months later, he increased his daily ingestion of DHEA to 50 mg with no adverse side effects. His level climbed slowly to 2.0, still low, with an optimum level reference of 1.5 to 7.0 mg/mL. He is also taking Saw Palmetto capsules to keep his prostate from swelling. Frank bumps his dosage of DHEA another 150 mg one hour before a heavy weight-resistance workout with noticeable strength and endurance spikes. These are all things that Dr. Anderson is monitoring closely, but by and large, DHEA causes very few negative side effects. DHEA certainly has been proven to be an adjunct, as we go forward in the quest for active health and longevity.

Human Growth Hormone (HGH)

HGH is a vital hormone which regulates the body's metabolism of proteins, carbohydrates, and electrolytes, and monitors the body's utilization of fat. HGH is secreted by the somotropic cells of the anterior lobe of the pituitary gland, at the base of the brain. HGH has been referred to as the Master Hormone, as it effects all the other endocrine glands and plays a major role in the growth and development of just about every organ in our body. While many hormones are secreted at a constant rate throughout the day, HGH is secreted in 15-minute pulses (not in a continuous stream) twice throughout a 24-hour period, with the major secretion occurring at night one to two hours after the onset of deep rapid eye movement (REM) sleep. Such sporadic occurrence indicates optimum supplementation of the hormone should be in tune with the body's circadian (24-hour) rhythm. Frank has determined his best results to occur when he administers 0.25 cc just before bedtime and 0.25 cc during the late hours of sleep when nature calls for a tap of his kidney. Younger recipients may need no more than 0.25 cc per night or alternate nights, depending on their IGF-I blood level, which we will discuss later. At the present time, pure HGH can only be administered subcutaneously, by injection. Frank's preferred site is the fat area at the sides of his waist, from which he has lost an astounding four inches of fatty tissue since beginning his HGH schedule.

Research has demonstrated strong connections between certain debilitating health conditions and the decline in HGH levels of older individuals. As we age and HGH secretions decrease, there is definite increase in total body weight, primarily body fat, together with a dramatic decrease in muscle and bone mass. These changes reduce strength, stamina and endurance, creating a noticeable loss of mental and physical energy. Also concomitant with a decrease in HGH is an increase in dangerous low-density lipoprotein and artery clogging triglycerides, thereby increasing the risk of heart disease and stroke, as well as creating an impaired sleep pattern and a weakened immune system; these debilitating conditions all lead to a reduction in the quality and longevity of life. Because of these findings, complementary physicians now consider aging as a treatable disease, the cause of which is due at least in part to the decline of our body's hormones, principally led by the HGH deficiency.

Interest in HGH for its anti-aging properties dates back to the early 1960's, when Vladimier Dillman, a Russian gerontologist, demonstrated that aging was directly related to a decline of our HGH production (Dillman, 1989). This research was then followed in 1989 by that of Dr. Jorgensen of Sweden who, using a double blind placebo controlled cross-over study, documented the benefits of HGH replacement therapy in aging adults with a noticeable increase in muscle mass, strength, and exercise stamina (Jorgensen, et al., 1994). In 1965, Dr. Allen Dunn, resident orthopathic surgeon at Cornell University Medical Center, took special note of acromegaly after-effects from over-secretion of Growth Hormone (GH) and deduced that supplementation, injected directly into osteoarthritic joints might promote joint repair and growth. His experiments on rabbits and dogs, injecting GH directly into degenerated joints resulted in 90% regeneration, impressive enough to encourage his patent of the method in 1994. Several complementary physicians have reported similar results in their human patients, but mainstream doctors are still skeptical about this revolutionary (we prefer to call it evolutionary) use of growth hormone to fight one of the post- prevalent debilitations of the normal aging process. Over 40 million Americans are plagued with arthritis, one in every seven of us. Frank has symptoms in his feet. Three mainstream physicians offered the same prescription to him for the pain he had been experiencing in his toes: 800 mg tablets of ibuprofen, the pain pill ingested like candy by the majority of America's aged arthritic citizens. The pill does alleviate the pain, but does not correct the condition. Too often, the mainstream prescription is a drug to mask pain, rather than try alternative nutritional adjustments or hormonal replacements that would alter the cause of pain. HGH may be the answer.

In July, 1990, the *New England Journal of Medicine* published an alarming report by Daniel Rudman and his colleagues at the Medical College of Wisconsin. Their research followed 12 elderly men who were given HGH for 6 months. The men lost 14.4% adipose tissue mass (visceral fat), while increasing their lean body mass (muscle) by 8.8%. The investigators concluded that "the effects of six months of supplemental HGH on lean body mass and adipose (fatty) tissue mass were equivalent in magnitude to the changes incurred during 10 to 20 years of aging."

During the last five years, hundreds of scientific studies have been conducted in England, Sweden, and Denmark, also documenting a long list of clinical improvements, including loss of body fat, gain in lean body mass, improved exercise performance, improved memory and cognition, improved lipid profiles, including lower LDL (bad cholesterol) and higher HDL (good cholesterol), and improved functioning of the immune system. Presently, complementary physicians are treating thousands of growth hormone-deficient patients with HGH supplementation. This practice should markedly increase, now that the FDA has approved HGH replacement therapy, because the cost has significantly decreased. Competition should drive the cost down markedly in the 21st century, when mainstream physicians recognize the benefits of this remarkable hormone.

In the 1997 issue of *Hospital Practice*, Silvio Inzucchi notes: "Growth hormone deficiency is now formally recognized as a specific clinical syndrome, typified by decreased muscle mass, increased body fat (predominantly at intra-abdominal sites), decreased exercise tolerance, osteopenia, abnormal lipid profiles, and diminished well-being." Treatment with HGH also shows promise in such adverse medical conditions as osteoporosis, obesity, heart failure, AIDS wasting, and acute catabolic illnesses. It is truly a serum from the Fountain of Youth.

Readers who consider HGH replacement must know their personal hormonal level which can be revealed by a simple blood test, measuring your IGF-1 (insulin-like growth factor). Normally, HGH is released into the blood stream for about 15 minutes twice a day, registering variable peaks and valleys, making it difficult to measure true total levels at any specific time. To obtain a more accurate measure of a person's current HGH level, we test for the principal product of HGH production, which is IGF-1, also called Somatomedin C. Frank's optimum range for his age of 67 is an IGF-I level of 71-290 mg/dl. At his first visit, his level was measured at 108. Four months after daily injection of only .5 IU's of HGH, his level rose to an astounding 232. He reported significant loss of visceral fat in the abdominal area, remarkable return of skin resilience with less wrinkling of the back of his hands, and hypertrophy of all the major muscle groups. Frank has tried to mimic his body's natural cycles and circadian rhythm. Because HGH is released in pulses and not a continuous stream (with the largest pulse coming at night during REM sleep), research has shown that the best time to administer HGH is by a subcutaneous injection at bedtime. REM is the time during sleep when dreams occur. Since Frank's night is usually disturbed by a call for urination (normal for senior patients who supplement their diets with vast amounts of micronutrients), he has split his daily dose in half, talking one-half before bedtime and the other after that nightly call at about 4:30 AM. His personal test comparisons have shown this regimen to be most efficacious.

In early trials of HGH therapy, some side effects were directly related to high dosage and frequency of HGH administration; these included elevated blood sugar levels, joint pain, and increased incidence of carpal tunnel syndrome (a painful condition of the wrist and hand). With continued research, however, we have learned that using small doses of HGH on a frequent basis, rather than large doses infrequently, almost entirely eliminates these side effects. The appropriate dosage for HGH varies from individual to individual, based on body composition, age, and physical needs. Therefore, of ultimate importance to our readers is finding a knowledgeable physician to assist in determining your optimum individualized dosages of HGH, which, along with your diet, supplements, and exercise, can end your quest for active health and longevity.

You may not want to go this far. You are probably tentative and cautious when it comes to accepting anti-aging theories. Who can blame you, when there is a plethora of conjecture in the longevity section of every book store? We repeat: We will not prescribe, but will only report our own progress. Our hunger for strength and vitality through the senior years is insatiable. We have, admittedly, been influenced by Plato, in his quest for the Perfect Form, and by other great teachers like Epicletus, the Greek stoic philosopher (55-135 A.D.) who wrote: "Tentative efforts lead to tentative outcomes Therefore, give yourself fully to your endeavors. Decide to construct your character through excellent actions and determine to pay the price of a worthy goal. The trials of your encounter will introduce you to your strengths. Remain steadfast… and one day you will build something that endures, something that is worthy of your potential." That something can be a strong and active physical countenance. The senior years that Frank has achieved already are energetic and powerful. His supplementation of HGH, in our opinion, will help to prolong them well into the next century. He is quite an anomaly in these years of the walking dead seniors.

Alternative Secretagogues

There is no longer doubt among complementary physicians, and certainly in the professional body-building community, that HGH supplementation will build muscle, stimulate energy, restore skin resilience, and nudge your gonads, but the cost is still high and many readers fear the needle. Seniors, you have no choice, since your IGF-1 level is probably quite low (be sure to have it tested before beginning an HGH supplementation program). Younger readers might consider "secretagogues," natural GH stimulants.

These growth hormone-releasing agents include amino acids such as arginine, omithine, lysine and glycine, which work synergistically to encourage your own pituitary gland to release growth hormone. Unfortunately, much of this GH cocktail would be destroyed by your low pH stomach acids, if you simply took these acids in pill form; little would reach your pituitary hypothalamus axis to cause secretion of HGH. Injection of a serum combining these acids might work, but then you are back to needles.

Recently, a "chaperone delivery system" was developed by Dr. James Jamieson to avoid the stomach acid degradation. The effervescent product developed by him delivers the growth hormone precursors in the form of pyroglytamate, shown to be more bioactive and to also contain somatostatin blockers. Somatostatin is an antagonistic compound that shuts down growth hormone receptors. Jamieson has reported increases between 8.5% and 36.6% of IGF-1 in body builders' blood tests after only 6 days of supplementation (*Ironman*, 1998). The GH product, called Symbiotropin, is available from a company called Muscle Linc at 1701 Ives Avenue, Oxnard, CA, 93033. Its over the counter version is called GH-STAK. Older readers might consider "stacking" this supplement with HGH injections to augment their effect, as Symbiotropin effectively blocks somatostatin with its "anterior pituitary peptides."

From SoCal Sports Supplements (1-800-667-6020) comes a similar product called GH Blast which boasts no "chaperone delivery system," but does include small amounts of glutamine, along with the secretagogues previously listed in the Symbiotropin. Glycine and glutamine are known neurotransmitter stimulants that affect the hypothalamus (our master control gland) encouraging GH secretion from the pituitary. This substance comes in powder form with a fruit punch flavor that suggests the inclusion of a high glycemic index sugar, probably included for insulin surge rapid transport into the bloodstream, before stomach acid degradation. It is worth considering, as a recent test by Dr. Dan Gwartney of Omaha, Nebraska, involving IGF-1 measurements of test recipients before and 90 minutes after ingestion of GH Blast reported an alarming average increase of 1271%. Blood levels of IGF-1, remember, are strong indicators of HGH secretion. If you believe in "considering the source", a wise caveat emptor for any investor, Gwartney pumps iron with high intensity and has developed a body of massive though sharply defined proportions, capable of scoring quite well in any body building competitive event. So Cal is at 565 Pearl Street, Suite 300, La Jolla, CA 92037. To counteract the problem of degradation by stomach acids from oral dosage, we suggest to chemists the development of a sublingual variety. Our suspicion is that other similar GH stimulants will be flooding the health food store shelves after the turn of the century, as new evidence of the efficacy of hormone replacement therapy brings us closer to the elusive Fountain of Youth.

As our book comes closer to publication, a hot communiqué from the professional world of body building has announced a new product from Meritech Pharmaceuticals, a genetic engineering corporation: Stabilized Sublingual Growth Hormone. The company claims it is the same substance we have been administering to ourselves by syringe, somatotropin, but their recombinant HGH is fed to the liver via droplets under the tongue (a sensitive door to the blood stream). Needle-phobics will welcome this news (and the tenth of the cost price tag), but Dr. Anderson is skeptical, since the Meritech product does not require a prescription. He suspects that it might be just another secretagogue, devised to stimulate secretion of HGH from the recipient's own pituitary gland. This reaction would indicate futile use of the product by older patients, as their own supply of HGH will have been naturally depleted. Younger patients may fare well, certainly welcoming the sublingual pathway in lieu of the needle.

Oral ingestion of HGH is contraindicated because of low pH stomach acids, which would render HGH inactive before it gets a chance to bind to the liver receptors that, in turn, secrete insulin growth factors. Meritech claims to have suspended their somatotropin and pituitary extract in an alcohol base. The alcohol is the principal carrier, transporting the HGH from the sensitive tissues under the tongue. The level of alcohol is high, 30x the somatotropin and 30x the pituitary extract, and 10 drops are prescribed, administered 3 times a day.

Meritech claims to have documented a 71% increase of IGF-1 production after only a short time of use, but has produced no double blind test results to back up their claim. We also wonder where they get their pituitary extract. Suffice to say that Meritech is to be commended for their foresight in developing a product that may boost 1GF-I levels, as elevation of IGF-I has been proven to result in the growth of muscle tissue. Surely, at the turn of the century, HGH will be more available at a much lower cost.

Whether you choose to supplement with the Meritech product sublingually or with humatrope via prescribed subcutaneous injection, we strongly advise you to boost your protein ingestion, as deficient protein consumption can hinder IGF-1 secretion, resulting in muscle catabolism (release of energy). HGH supplementation with no indicated rise of IGF-1 levels will catabolize muscle. This result will happen if your protein consumption is low. This state has been observed among body builders who fast to look “more defined” at contest time.

Optimum protein consumption is dependent upon your level of physical exertion. If that level is close to zero, the Recommended Daily Allowance (RDA) standards apply to you. If you follow a program of exercise, such as we present for you later in this book, those standards are far from adequate. Forget the RDA standards if you are training with weights at high intensity. Their standards will barely keep you alive (have you witnessed the anorexic countenance of most vegetarians?), but they are certainly insufficient to build and sustain muscle. For a body builder to remain in a positive nitrogen balance (ideal for protein synthesis), he must ingest between 1 and 2 grams of protein per pound of his body weight. Champions are ingesting between 300 and 500 gm of protein a day. IGF-1 levels have been documented to decrease after several days of fasting, despite HGH supplementation. If you plan to take HGH either by injection or sublingually, be sure to keep your protein ingestion high or you will defeat your purpose.

Changes that co-author Frank has experienced from HGH supplementation include renewed skin resilience (after just 3 weeks), a 25% rise in his high-density lipoprotein, 100% increase in his IGF-1 level, 25% drop in triglycerides, and a 100% increase in his DHEA level (all after only 3 months). This rise in DHEA may be partly due to his additional supplementation of this vital prohormone (available over the counter). Frank’s testosterone was sluggish, however, until a shot of testosterone cypionate every 10 days boosted his level to that of a 20-year-old, which it held for a few months. This boost could account for a soaring of his strength quotient and an annoying preoccupation with sex, but frequent visits to the health clubs and an understanding wife have relieved those anxieties. Gratifying was the drop of Frank's total cholesterol count from 284 to its current 157, despite his periodic ingestion of his favorite breakfast of four eggs over-medium plus two orders of crisp bacon. Eggs have taken a bad rap. They have never been responsible for elevating cholesterol. With lecithin dominating the yolk of eggs as a cholesterol emulsifier, eggs just might be one of our most perfect foods. Frank's currently low cholesterol number may be due in part to a doubling of his Phosphatidyl Choline, niacin, garlic, cayenne and ayur guggulipid, all recommended by Dr. Anderson in lieu of common drug treatments for high cholesterol prescribed by mainstream physicians.

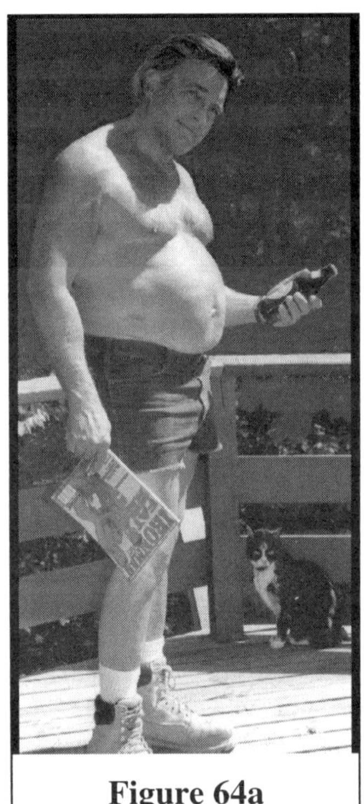

Figure 64a

Frank, appearing six months pregnant, prior to his first visit with Dr. Anderson.

Most noticeable, since Frank began to supplement with HGH, is an increase of hard, lean muscle tissue, a fast depletion of fat around his waist, and a welcome enhancement of mental function. He is presently completing two new books while delivering week-long classical art seminars to semi-professional artists nationwide, but he still finds time to teach downhill skiing to guests of his wife's bed and breakfast in Vermont. Frank has personally helped students to produce over 17,500 paintings in the past 35 years, most of them portraits. Although diversified, these interests have a common denominator: To preserve classical tradition against the formidable modern aberrations of art and skiing that are currently in vogue. It takes strength to be a dinosaur when the species is nearly extinct, but there are a sufficient number of artists still enamored with the classical manner of painting and

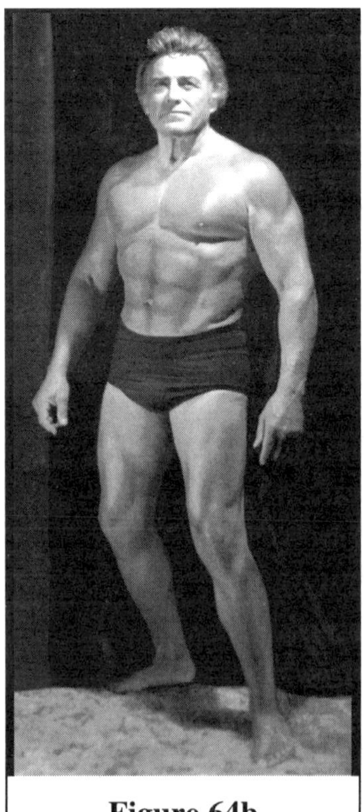

Figure 64b

Frank 12 months later

enough skiers who still appreciate the elegance of the Austrian form of the late fifties to keep Frank busy.

None of these activities would be possible without a healthy countenance, though, perpetuated by religious attendance at health clubs, a high-protein diet and vitamin, mineral and antioxidant supplementation. The HGH regimen has rekindled his energy to youthful levels. Most 67-year-old men would find it difficult to lift Frank's luggage. He will be 68 years old when this book is published. Frank is planning to switch to the HGH sublingual form soon, to see if this new Meritech product can keep his IGF-1 level elevated. We would like to provide another book for you in 30 years, when Frank approaches 100, informing you of his progress. For now, we urge you to compare his countenance, prior to his first visit to Dr. Anderson (Fig. 64a), to his silhouette only twelve months later (Fig. 64b); when you do, we have little doubt that you will want to continue reading about our *Rage Against Age*.

Pregnenolone

As we mentioned in the previous chapter, DHEA is the mother hormone. Pregnenolone is considered by many to the grandmother or parent hormone, as it is the precursor to DHEA, and therefore, to estrogen, testosterone and other natural steroid pathways. Like DHEA, pregnenolone is produced in the brain, where it is found in high concentrations, as well as in the adrenal glands. Like most of the hormones in the body, we know that the production of pregnenolone, as with other hormones, declines drastically with age. Rates of decline vary from person to person, but, by the time you are into your fourth decade, there is a tremendous decrease in pregnenolone production.

Pregnenolone is the hormone that is key to keeping our brains functioning at their peak capacity; some researchers believe that it is the most potent memory enhancer. Even more exciting is that pregnenolone enhances our ability to perform on the job while heightening our feelings of well-being, psychic energy, joie de vivre, fighting mental fatigue, improving memory, relieving depression, and also enhances our mood. It's a natural equivalent to a caffeine/Prozac cocktail.

One interesting fact about pregnenolone is that it had been identified back in the 1940's, and, at that time, was quite successful as a treatment for rheumatoid arthritis. Because it was a hormone produced inside our bodies, it was not able to be patented, and therefore, was overshadowed by the discovery of the synthetic cortisones, from which huge profits could be earned. Today, in addition to enhancement of our mental function, pregnenolone is being studied for use in treating Alzheimer's disease, as well as for the treatment of multiple sclerosis, spinal cord injuries, cardiovascular problems, bolstering the immune system, and for strengthening the integrity of the collagen in the skin. Recent studies performed both on rats and mice proved mental enhancement through the use of small doses of pregnenolone. Human studies on airline pilots showed their mental capacities in flight simulators were markedly improved with exposure to pregnenolone, even in small doses. Pregnenolone is available, over the counter, at any reputable health produce store at a reasonable cost.

As with DHEA, pregnenolone levels can be determined from a patient's blood, drawn and monitored at the lab. Most people require somewhere between 20 to 50 mg of supplementation on a daily basis. Frank has been supplementing 50 mg daily for one year. His current blood level is still low, indicating a need to increase his daily dosage; Dr. Anderson has advised him to double it. As you consider the mental and anti-aging benefits of pregnenolone, you may want your complementary physician to put a dosage into your supplementation program.

Estrogen

Estrogen, as we all know, is predominantly a female hormone that regulates a woman's maturation process from menarche, through fertility, and eventually, menopause; lower levels are found, surprisingly, in men. Similar to the declines we have described in our other super-hormone observations, a woman's estrogen levels begin to fall when she reaches her forties, nose-diving in her early fifties. Girls average estradiol blood levels of 200 picograms per milliliter; that level drops to an average of 30 pc/ml after menopause. In women, estrogen is produced in the ovaries and adrenal glands, while in men, a small amount is produced only in the adrenal glands from testosterone. Women also produce some testosterone in their ovaries and adrenal glands. Female body builders often supplement their diet with testosterone precursors to boost their level and promote massive masculine musculature. Why they would want bodies that look masculine is puzzling, but may be indicative of hormonal imbalance. The preponderance of one or the other hormones determines the sexual characteristic of an individual during fetal development. Anomalies occur, and lower levels of gender specific hormones could influence sexual preference after puberty.

Before discussing the importance of estrogen hormone replacement as female anti-aging therapy, let us look at the various types of estrogen found in a woman's body and explore what would be the safest yet effective forms to use for its replacement.

Three types of estrogen are produced in a woman's body: estrone, estradiol, and estriol; all are regulated by the hypothalamus, just above the pituitary gland. Estrone is the strongest, estradiol is somewhat weaker, and estriol is the weakest. Although estrogen is not a carcinogen, stronger estrogens are apt to stimulate tumor growth because estrogen is trophic, a growth hormone. Therefore, complementary physicians prefer to use weaker forms which have less carcinogenic potential but are still effective. Estrogen alone can cause hyperplasia (excessive growth of the endometrium, the uterus lining). Hyperplasia is recognized as a precursor to cancer. Paradoxically, estrogen is a potent antioxidant, a strong defender against free radical invaders.

The pros and cons of using Estrogen Replacement Therapy, "The Estrogen Dilemma" (*TIME*, June 26, 1995), has been a hot medical issue for the last 25 years because of a paradox, fueled and confused by the fact that the estrogen most commonly used by mainstream physicians for hormone replacement therapy for the last 25 years is not the same in chemical structure as the estrogen produced in a woman's body. Their preferred synthetic version is a blend of different types of estrogen found in the urine of pregnant mares, marketed for years under the brand name Premarin. Premarin is stronger than the estrogen produced naturally in a woman's body (Notelovitz, "Estrogen Replacement Therapy: Indications, Contraindications, and Agent Selection", *American Journal of Obstetrics and Gynecology*, 1989).

The estrogen form more commonly used by alternative or complementary physicians is called Biest or Triest. Biest is a combination of 80% estriol, which, as you remember is the weakest form of estrogen, and 20% estradiol. Triest is a combination of 80% estriol, 10% estradiol, and 10% estrone. Research has shown that estriol has a protective effect against breast cancer and in fact, appears to inhibit tumor growth. Also it has been documented that women with breast cancer have lower-than-normal levels of estriol and higher levels of estrone. Another problem that existed for years in traditional medicine was that estrogen was supplemented alone, without concurrent use of a natural companion female hormone, progesterone; this also increased the risk of breast and uterine cancer, as well as creating an unnatural hormonal imbalance. Considerable research within the last five years, has encouraged most traditional physicians to use a combination of Premarin and progesterone for supplemental replacement. The pharmaceutical giants responded with Prempro, a combined medication, using Premarin plus a synthetic progesterone. Skeptical about the necessity of equine involvement, alternative or complementary physicians prefer using Triest or Biest as the estrogen, combining it with Progestin, a natural progesterone developed from diosgenin, a compound found in the wild yam, for synergistic female hormone therapy with no carcinogenic side effects and with excellent results.

Beyond virtually eliminating the symptoms of menopause, estrogen and progesterone replacement offers many other anti-aging benefits. The two hormones are important for maintaining a strong immune system, resulting in a healthy body that prevents disease and debilitation; Estrogen Replacement Therapy (ERT) preserves youthful resilience. ERT has been proven to protect or greatly reduce the risk of osteoporosis by slowing down the rate of bone loss, preserving a woman's strength and mobility. Progesterone has been observed by Jerilynn C. Prior of the University of British Columbia in Vancouver to stimulate osteoblasts (reconstructive bone cells) to form new bone. Women taking estrogen with progesterone have a 25% reduction in bone loss, and only one-fourth the number of hip fractures. Spine fractures and tooth loss are also decreased by 50%. Many incidents of tooth separation are related to progesterone deficiency. California physician Dr. John R. Lee defines osteoporosis as one result of the natural decline of this hormone.

ERT reduces the risk of heart disease, including heart attack from arterial constriction, stroke, congestive heart failure, and arrhythmia. Research has shown that heart disease is rare in pre-menopausal women, increasing three-fold, however, during the post-menopausal years due to the decline in levels of estrogen (Stampfer, et al., "Post-menopausal Estrogen Therapy and Cardiovascular Disease", *New England Journal of Medicine*, 1992). ERT dilates and relaxes the arteries. Women who use estrogen replacement have half the risk of developing heart disease, because estrogen strengthens both the heart muscles and blood vessels, as well as lowers LDL levels, while it raises HDL levels.

ERT sharpens a woman's thinking, enhances their mood and may prevent Alzheimer's disease. The discovery of estrogen receptors in the brain explains why women's brains seem to work differently than men's. It has been speculated that most men respond well to spatial challenges, while women are better mathematical calculators, although Frank has witnessed quite the reverse in the academic art classes he conducts. So much for speculation.

Fluctuating hormone levels seem to have such a powerful effect on the mood of women and may explain why one of the symptoms of menopause is severe depression. Women using estrogen replacement reported an overall elevation of mood and a greater sense of well-being. Also, women who have used estrogen therapy are less likely to develop Alzheimer's disease, because estrogen is involved in the formation and protection of brain cells, indirectly triggering the production of a key neurotransmitter that is essential to the memory function of our brain.

ERT will restore or rejuvenate sexual desire and pleasure. Most women experience some degree of vaginal thinning after menopause due to estrogen loss. If this declining level of estrogen is not supplemented, the vaginal walls thin out, and there is a decline in the production of the secretions that lubricate the vagina, resulting in the vaginal tissue becoming less pliable, making sexual intercourse uncomfortable, and soon, undesirable.

ERT improves skin quality, resulting in fewer wrinkles. Estrogen replacement "rounds out" a woman's body, softening her skin, increasing or maintaining male-attracting body fat as is found in the breasts and buttocks. ERT also maintains or improves muscle tone, which helps keep skin from sagging and becoming wrinkled. There is no doubt that ERT, like HGH, is an elixir poured directly from the Fountain of Youth. By encouraging women to use estrogen and progesterone as a part of their total hormone replacement program, we can safely and effectively assure many long-term female benefits that can lead to their active health and longevity.

For the small percentage of women who cannot tolerate the side effects that a few experience from ERT (diabetics often experience a worsening of their condition as do some hypertensive patients), large doses of folic acid and boron have been reported by Dr. Atkins to restore menstrual regularity and adjust hormonal imbalances. Boron is a mineral necessary to retain bone density in post-menstrual women. He recommends 3-8 mg of this vital supplement for everyone. Vitamin E supplementation will ease hot flashes and stimulate vaginal secretions, often eliminating the need for hysterectomy. In addition, we advise women with any of the following conditions to consider alternatives to ERT:

- History or presence of breast cancer

- Pregnancy or imminent anticipation of pregnancy
- Thrombophlebitis (inflammation of the veins)
- Undiagnosed abnormal vaginal bleeding
- Stroke
- Liver disease
- A desire to win the Ms. Olympia Bodybuilding Contest. Contestants wishing to please the judges have no choice but to reject ERT and adopt TRT (Testosterone Replacement Therapy), guaranteed to produce the muscular countenance of a man. But, why, girls... why?

Progesterone

Progesterone is a female sex hormone produced in the corpus luteum (the follicle that ruptures during ovulation), the adrenal glands, and in the placenta during pregnancy. Progesterone plays a major role in the menstrual cycle, as it prepares the uterine lining to accept the egg if it is fertilized. If there is no fertilization, progesterone levels drop, triggering the sloughing off of the lining of the uterus. Progesterone is also vital to a healthy pregnancy, and, without sufficient progesterone, a woman has a difficult time carrying her pregnancy full term.

As a woman approaches her thirties, her progesterone levels begin to decline and her menopausal discomfort, hot flashes and mood swings are due to the lack of balance between estrogen and progesterone. In addition, progesterone plays an important role in many body functions:

- Controls a woman's sex drive, enhances the sex drive women sometimes feel during ovulation, promoting a feeling of well-being.
- Halts the progression of osteoporosis and in fact, stimulates osteoblasts to form new bone. Dr. John Lee, in his book titled, *Natural Progesterone*, states that progesterone is probably responsible for healthy bones, since bone mass begins decreasing at the same age when progesterone levels begin to drop.
- An effective treatment for certain nerve diseases, such as multiple sclerosis, as it promotes the formation of the myelin sheath, the fatty substance that surrounds and protects nerve fibers.

As with estrogen, which we discussed earlier, there is also a synthetic progesterone, Progestin, which alternative physicians have used for years. In fact, many mainstream physicians are not aware of the significant differences between progesterone, Progestin, estrogen and Premarin. Synthetic hormones are man-made chemicals that resemble the molecular structure that the body normally produces. Natural hormone replacement supplements resemble molecularly and chemically the hormones found in our bodies, and therefore, cannot be patented for profit from sales, so the pharmaceutical industry has no interest in marketing them. When you add progesterone to your hormone replacement protocol, ask your doctor or an alternative physician about the availability of natural progesterone; it probably will cost less, and your body will respond to it more effectively.

Testosterone

Testosterone is the principal hormone responsible for male sexual development during puberty, characteristics like pubic hair growth, penile erections and nocturnal emissions, deeper voice, thickening of the skin and increased bone density. Man's energy level, mood, libido, sperm production, strength and aggression are all directly related to his specific level of testosterone, which arouses man's passion, gusto and "eye of the tiger." Like all the hormones we have discussed so far, men's testosterone levels decline rapidly with age. Between the age of the late thirties and his mid-forties, man's aging clock in his brain signals that it is time for his testosterone levels to decline. As the estrogen of women in menopause diminishes, there is a gradual decline of testosterone in men, accelerating with each passing year. This degeneration or change in a man's life has been called male menopause, andropause, or age-related testosterone decline, more rapid in the physically inactive, indicating a relationship between T production and heavy physical activity. Computer nerds can expect a rapid decline of this masculine hormone.

Whatever you wish to call it, the decline of free testosterone, which is the biologically active testosterone, is very common with aging and can have dramatic consequences. The impact of decreased testosterone levels in man can present itself with a progressive decrease in energy, mild depression with increased irritability, thinning bone muscle atrophy, increased body fat (especially in the midsection of his body), and impaired sexual function. Since he also carries a level of the female hormone, the physically inactive senior male will take on female characteristics, like a higher voice, a softer body, a pear shape, and a sweeter, more gentle personality. Perhaps you know some retired senior men who fit this profile; they are legion.

Knowing all that we do about male menopause or andropause, why is testosterone not being replaced in men with this hormone deficiency? Why is TRT so far behind ERT for women, which has been in existence for more than 20 years? One of Frank's senior students, a Texas nurse who had been exposed to estrogen replacement for several years, confessed to him that her doctor had mentioned the availability of testosterone for her progressively more delicate husband, but Beverly asked the physician to keep quiet about it, as she was enjoying the absence of aggressive behavior that had been her husband's macho manner for so many years.

Men, in general, are not comfortable discussing the symptoms of testosterone deficiency with friends or coworkers, let alone their wives or girlfriends, or even their family physician. Many men would rather suffer quietly the decline of masculinity they are experiencing and rationalize it as a normal characteristic of "getting older." Few seek professional help. Unlike female menopause which is heralded by cessation of periods, hot flashes, and mood changes, male andropause does not have any obvious specific physiological markers to announce its arrival. The onset of symptoms in many men can be insidious. Notably, the male body building community has been responsible for much of our medical knowledge in this area; as its professionals have been using steroidal TRT for over two decades to build Herculean physiques (some to the point of excessive abuse). Mainstream medical conjecture is often dependent upon the results of double blind tests administered to rats, mice, and rabbits. Medical researchers are reluctant to deduce from human experimentation, due to our increasingly litigious society. Retired champion body builders who have shrunk remarkably from cessation of TRT have also proven that termination of TRT will result in the "normal" resumption of testosterone decline with its concomitant diminishment of masculinity and, in our opinion, acceleration of the aging process.

Better testosterone precursors taken orally by "natural " body builders all include the herb Saw Palmetto. For years, many physicians had concerns about administering TRT with fear that high levels would increase the chances of men getting prostate cancer. In the last three years, research between 1995 and 1998 at Johns Hopkins, as well as Baylor University, has been able to document that high levels of testosterone do not increase the risk of prostate cancer. Prostate size may increase, but this change can be controlled with supplementation of Saw Palmetto and Pygeum, two natural herbs that probably kept Primitive Man's prostate from enlarging. When Frank's PSA indicated enlargement, probably from his new regimen of testosterone precursors, we were able to lower it five points simply by boosting his supplementation of these two herbs. The excitement surrounding HRT with testosterone comes from the growing realization that many of the symptoms men have come to accept as a normal part of the aging process are likely due to the decline of their testosterone levels; TRT can correct this hormonal imbalance.

In addition to improving strength, energy, sexual function and overall body composition, periodic supplemental testosterone injection helps the heart remain healthy. In a study at Columbia Medical School, Dr. G. Phillips found that lower testosterone levels accompanied high incidence and severity of heart disease. Supplemental testosterone appears to raise the good cholesterol (HDL) and lower the bad cholesterol (LDL), thus sweeping the arterial walls of plaque with a profound preventive effect against heart disease.

As we mentioned earlier, women also have small amounts of testosterone that are produced by their ovaries. When a woman approaches menopause, along with her estrogen and progesterone levels, her testosterone level also drops. If her testosterone is not at its optimal level, despite hormone replacement with Estrogen and Progesterone, the female body may still be out of balance, causing a notable decline in a woman's libido. In addition to boosting a woman's libido, testosterone supplementation enhances the functions of estrogen and progesterone in strengthening bones and preventing osteoporosis.

A few years ago, one of Dr. Anderson's patients was a lovely woman in her 40's who had a total hysterectomy in her early 30's due to excessive bleeding from fibroids. Her OB/GYN physician started her on Premarin shortly after her surgery, but when Dr. Anderson met her in her mid-forties, she had gained weight (18 lbs.) and had no sexual interest whatsoever. These problems were obviously of great concern to her and her husband of seven years. The doctor advised mild testosterone supplementation and gave her some literature to read that he could then review with her on her next visit. At that visit, she decided to try the testosterone supplement, which was supplied in a cream form to be applied to the skin on any part of her body. About three weeks later she returned to report things were definitely improved, and, for the first time in a long time, she actually initiated foreplay, which eventually led to intercourse. Four weeks following that visit, both she and her husband came in to tell Dr. Anderson what a remarkable difference the testosterone supplement had made in their relationship. Since then, he has been able to help numerous women have more complete and satisfied libido than they have had in years.

Of course, when we talk about TRT, we are not promoting the abuse of excess testosterone supplementation for "bulking up" young body builders who already have their normal supply. We advise replacement of the hormone only for those men and women whose levels have drastically declined. Your personal level can easily be determined by standard blood analysis. For men and women, boosting testosterone to youthful levels can demonstrate the dramatic difference between living a senior life of depression and weakness with chronic fatigue, and leading a strong, passionate and healthy aged life with masculine and feminine vigor. The effects can be accelerated, of course, if you combine TRT with a program of progressive weight-resistance exercise, interrupted sporadically with aerobic activity and daily doses of HGH. Frank Covino is living proof of this rejuvenating process. The Fountain of Youth is thus within your reach. We fervently believe that this book has led you there. Whether you drink from this well is up to you and your complementary physician. You are now in control of your own destiny.

Testosterone and Nandrolone Precursors (Anabolic Prohormones)

While DHEA has been defined by us as a safe oral testosterone precursor, supplemented in proper dosage (as determined by your blood test level) and enhanced by its mother hormone, pregnenolone, its conversion to testosterone can be blocked by a process called aromatase, steering it toward an estrogen pathway. Men are strongly advised to include flavone supplementation to inhibit estrogen conversion when beginning DHEA supplementation. The best flavone currently available, although it has only been proven to work in a test tube, is a product called Chrysin, which offers the phytochemicals protodioscin and furostanol. They synergistically suppress estrogen, actually lowering its level. All the products listed in this segment are natural products, thus unpatentable, and available in any health store with informed personnel.

Advanced body builders are leading the way for older men whose testosterone levels have nose-dived. They are ingesting a prohormone that is closer in line to testosterone production than DHEA; it is called androstenedione, naturally produced by the adrenal gland. But, as we have revealed elsewhere, the adrenals get sluggish as the years pass, and the precursors diminish along with testosterone. Supplementation of androstenedione has proven to raise testosterone levels over 300%, but this jolt only seems to last two hours. For this reason, a timed release androstenedione product should be sought for constant efficacy.

East German Olympians were supposed to have used a nasal spray of "Andro," decidedly increasing their strength and stamina rapidly, because of the receptivity of the nose's sensitive, internal tissue. German Democratic Republic swimmer Raik Hannemann boasted that androstenedione was "mandatory for any athlete who wanted to compete in the 1988 Seoul Olympics." Be forewarned, however, that Andro in excess is still subject to aromatase possibilities that can steer the hormone toward an estrogen pathway. Some professional body builders have contracted female characteristics like gynecomastia (breast tissue), which can only be removed by surgery. Other negative side effects reported are hair loss and acne. Wise men who ingest this supplement take an estrogen buffer like Chrysin to guard against these unpleasant reactions. On the plus side, only one 50 mg oral dose of androstenedione will raise a man's testosterone level 150% (reported by German patent #DE 42 14 953 A 1), albeit for the short duration of two hours.

Chemist Derek Cornelius of Syntrax Innovations, USA, has found a more potent anabolic prohormone that boosts testosterone production with few, if any, side effects. This hormone is labeled 19-Norandrostenedione, now an essential supplement available to all natural body builders who crave maximum strength and size without use of injectable steroid. The hormone is three times more effective than Andro, with few noticeable side effects considered undesirable. Lacking a carbon atom at the 19th position, instead of converting to testosterone, 19-Norandrostenedione takes a direct path to the liver and converts to Nandrolone decanoate, a twin to the injectable steroid, Deca-Durabolin. This steroid was the most popular anabolic choice of professional body builders, prior to 1990, when drug tests were begun to discourage abuse of anabolic steroids. Extremely anabolic when combined with heavy-weight resistance, Nandrolone remains active much longer than Testosterone. Deca was the most widely used steroid in the 1980's, explaining why the body-building profession of that decade took such a giant leap forward in the cultivation of rock-hard, superhuman muscle and visible vascularity. In addition, Deca-Durabolin was proven to heal joint inflammation and lure pain away from stressed tendons. With no possibility of aromatasation, Deca is actually safer than Testosterone, producing the same anabolic effects with far less androgenic side effects. Deca, however, is currently illegal, banned by the

FDA. 19-Noarandrostenedione is a naturally occurring Nandrolone-producing prohormone that can be found advertised in any current physical culture magazine which appeals to serious body builders who are interested in developing their full body potential without injecting dangerous drugs. There are several over-the-counter (OTC) products that include it. Timed release is again preferred, as all prohormones have a short half life. A constant trickle of any precursor is better than a quickly expended gush. On the shelf of Vites and Herbs Sports Shoppe in Williston, Vermont, recently I was surprised to find a sublingual variety of 19-Norandrostenedione, which the manufacturer claims will enter the blood stream much faster than the orally administered tablet. 19-Norandrostenedione is converted to Nandrolone by the enzyme 17-beta-hydroxy-steroid dehydrogenase at a rate of 5.6%.

One of the major concerns about boosting testosterone levels is that excess testosterone can bind to dehydrotestosterone (DHT) and lead to prostate enlargement. Cornelius kept searching for a prohormone that could stimulate testosterone production without binding to DHT and found one which also interferes with estrogen production at the receptor level. Called 5-androstenediol, its 17-alphs alkylated version has been used by informed body builders for years under the anabolic steroid name, Methandriol. However, Methandriol is an injectable drug, currently illegal under FDA regulations. 5-androstenediol is a legal OTC oral twin to Methandriol, sometimes referred to as Pentabol and is also a potent anti-catabolic substance, since it protects against cortisol attacks on proteinaceious tissue. This substance is highly recommended for men with low testosterone levels, who wish to avoid injecting Testosterone Cypionate as a booster.

Writing for the hard-core muscle-building magazine called *MuscleMag International*, professional body builder Greg Zulak is highly respected for his honest evaluation of anabolic products. While he cannot legally prescribe steroids for muscular development, he bravely reveals the chemical stacks used by body building champions, that, together with high-intensity, weight-resistant exercise, has created their gargantuan physiques. Greg agrees with my description of 5-andro as an orally administered OTC product that mimics the steroid Methandriol, but he goes farther and labels it less effective than the 4-andro variation.

The numbers refer to the carbon position where testosterone and nortestosterone double-bond. The double-bond actually occurs at the 4th carbon position, but chemists find it more expensive to produce 4-androstenedione and

4-androstenediol products, hence the cheaper 5-Andro combination in products like Anotesten, commendably time-released, which I have tried and can attest to its effectiveness. Afraid of litigation because of its relationship to steroids, many U.S. health food stores refuse to stock Anotesten. As noted elsewhere, we will not prescribe, but it surely is a nuisance for me to have to call 1-800-246-3261 every time I run out of this anabolic product.

4- and 5- Andro prohormones certainly work, but as fast as I could write that last sentence, a new product is about to stir the prohormone industry. This new product will pale the effectiveness of 4- and 5- Andro, converting to Nandrolone three time faster than 19-Norandrostenedione, via the enzyme 3-beta-hydrosysteroid dehydrogenase. More anti-catabolic than any other precursor, 19-Noarandrostenediol will blow away all its competition. Taken in combination with 19-Norandrostenedione, preferably time released, body builders can now experience steroid effects (compounded Nandrolone) with avoidance of the needle. The converting enzymes are constant, however, capable of converting a set amount of prohormone at each ingestion. Any excess precursor could possibly convert to estrogen via aromatasation, but most will be excreted in the urine following metabolism. Safeguarding against the former side effect with a flavone-like Chrysin would be wise, as would the inclusion of Saw Palmetto to guard against the possibility of DHT binding and prostate enlargement.

19-Norandrostenediol does not only build muscle, but also regulates systemic resistance against many lethal infections, including pancreopathy and virus-caused myocardiopathy 100 times more effectively than DHEA. Like phosphatidyl serine, 19-Norandrostenediol protects against glucocorticoids which are known to suppress the immune system, preventing cytokine production and the proliferation of lymphocytes. Connective tissue, venous tissue and muscle tissue are all susceptible to glucocorticoid attack.

All things considered, weight-resistance exercise and the stacked daily ingestion of the supplements 19-Norandrostenedione with 19-Norandrostenediol, Saw Palmetto, Chrysin, and phosphatidyl choline is a positive step men can take against the aging process. Such a regimen can halt and raise the natural decline of testosterone, avoiding "andropause" and the diseases that seem to occur concurrent to its diminshment. Older men may still require the faster route of Testosterone Cypionate injection, if their testosterone count has hit rock bottom. Readers are advised to have their testosterone level checked. Women, too. Your level is probably lower than you think!

Hormone replacement therapy, together with testosterone prohormone or precursor supplementation, will be an important weapon in men's rage against age, as we enter the 21st century. Women can come along for the ride with ERT and low doses of DHEA. It is our opinion that this cutting-edge technology will build a superhuman variation of our species in the next several decades, increasing life expectancy and possibly extending what we now accept as our maximum life span. Stay tuned to the latest developments by subscribing to the best current physical culture magazines and discussing the new natural products they promote with your complementary physician. The mainstream medical establishment is reluctant to experiment on human patients, but have learned a lot from the self-sacrificing professional body-building community. So have we, as nutritional and ergogenic supplements are speeding us toward the destination of active longevity. Get on board now. It's going to be one helluva ride!

Melatonin

Melatonin is the primary neurohormone, both manufactured and secreted by the pineal gland located at the base of the brain. Unlike many other hormones in the body which are cholesterol-based, melatonin consists of a chain of amino acids. Melatonin is made from the amino acid tryptophan, which is an essential amino acid, found in meat, poultry, pumpkin seeds, sunflower seeds, baked potato skins and bananas. Once tryptophan is ingested, the body converts it into the neurotransmitter serotonin, which at night then becomes converted to melatonin.

The production of melatonin stops at sunrise and begins at sunset, thereby controlling the body's clock, or circadian rhythm, of the sleep-wake cycle. Changes in light are the key to secretion of melatonin. Light suppresses the release of melatonin, but as sunset begins, the dimming light transferred through the retina of the eyes into the pineal gland stimulates the release of more melatonin. The levels of melatonin peak from midnight to two in the morning, thus stimulating a greater quality of sleep or a greater amount of deep REM sleep, which is the most restorative and invigorating for the body.

At birth, and as we age toward puberty or pre-puberty, our melatonin levels rise. At puberty, there is a big drop in melatonin, which some believe is responsible for the first stages of puberty in both males and females. This drop could partly account for teenagers wanting to stay up all night. Subsequently, the levels of melatonin continue to drop linearly with age. As we know, sleep disorders are more common in the elderly, meaning the sleep-wake cycle is not being regulated as well, and they are not getting the quality of sleep they need.

Research has also documented that melatonin supplementation reduces the time needed to fall asleep, promotes vivid dreaming, reduces the number of times people awaken at night, and unlike prescription drugs, does not have next day "hangover effects" or addictive potential. Thus, for years, melatonin has been used among many "jet-setters" to treat the well-documented condition known as jet lag. Frank flies over 100,000 miles a year to deliver classical art seminars. At the age of 67, this nationwide schedule necessitates a sleep regulator like melatonin, which is the first thing he packs before a trip.

Beyond the regulation of our sleep-wake cycle, through research by Regelson and Pierpaoli in their book called, *The Melatonin Miracle,* and Dr. Regelson's book called, *The Superhormone Promise*, we have learned of the many benefits of melatonin as an anti-aging agent, a restorer of sexual rejuvenation, a booster to our immune system, and of its cancer-fighting power due to its powerful antioxidant properties. Because the focus of this book is on aging, we will concentrate on the anti-aging benefits of melatonin, but our readers are advised to thoroughly research this important hormone. Presently, we know that at about the age of 45 the pineal gland appears to slow down, and melatonin secretion levels markedly decline, which has a domino effect on other hormones that communicate with melatonin. Subsequently, the functioning of our body systems also slow down, and we recognize the symptoms of what is known as aging. In their research, Pierpaoli and Regelson "traded" the pineal glands of four month old mice (approximately teenagers) with those of 24-month-old mice (approximately 65 to 70 human years). The young mice with the old pineal glands began to age very rapidly, noted by changes in hair and skin quality, and by decreased energy. They died 30% earlier that the control mice. Conversely, young pineal glands transplanted in older mice created mice with improved quality of fur, plus a remarkable increase in energy. They lived 30% longer than expected.

Such experiments like this opened the door for learning about other hormones and their anti-aging benefits. If the decrease in melatonin is one of the natural events responsible for aging, then we, theoretically, could delay aging by restoring the hormone back to its healthy level. We are thus capable of "turning back the clock." Aging is no longer an inevitable physical condition, but can now be identified as a disease that can be treated and cured with adequate supplementation of vital hormones. Because melatonin, DHEA, pregnenolone and the Andro products are new, your mainstream doctor will probably not approve of their use. It may be irrelevant that these products are made from natural foods, are cheap, and available at any health food store, thus depriving him of profit from a prescription or pharmaceutical kickback. Our recommendations are based upon the results we have witnessed in many patients and bodybuilding colleagues.

Osteoporosis

Osteoporosis is a progressive and debilitating disease, characterized by low bone mass and deterioration of bone tissue, resulting in weak bones prone to fracture.

The risk of developing osteoporosis increases with age, as your peak bone mass is reached at age 35. Poor diet with insufficient calcium to meet your body's requirements is the main cause of osteoporosis, along with decreased levels of estrogen and progesterone, as well as lack of weight-resistant exercise, resulting in a gradual loss of bone mass. Osteoporosis affects primarily women, because their bone mass is 30% less than the bone mass of men. Thanks to osteoporosis, Americans suffer over one million broken bones a year. Of women over 45, one of four have some degree of osteoporosis, and nine of ten women over the age of 75 have it.

For women, the most rapid rate of bone loss occurs in the first five years after menopause, beginning around the age of 45. Women can virtually lose 5% to 10% of their bone mass during this period. The rate of bone loss then drops to about 1% a year. Men do not experience bone loss until after age 70, but once they do contract osteoporosis, the condition can be quite severe. Risk factors that enhance predisposition include:

- Inadequate nutrition—The popular American diet of processed food, carbonated soft drinks, caffeine, and excessive sugar and salt consumption can promote osteoporosis.
- Early menopause—Menopause-related osteoporosis is generally attributed to a lack of estrogen, but the major hormone deficiency of concern is progesterone. Before menopause actually begins, the body starts to decrease its output of progesterone. Bones slowly begin to lose their mass even prior to menopause. When menstruation ceases, osteoporosis accelerates because estrogen levels fall, and the already-decreasing bone mass is even more rapidly depleted.

- Smoking—Cigarette smoking appears to promote osteoporosis by inhibiting estrogen's effect on osteoblast cells and by lowering estrogen concentration in the blood stream. Hampered breathing because of smoking prevents carbon dioxide from exiting the body, as normally happens in an exhaled breath. Carbon dioxide retention leads to higher blood levels of carbonic acid, which the body attempts to neutralize with calcium from bones.
- Broad spectrum antibiotics—Abuse of antibiotic use can often deplete normal intestinal flora that supply the body with vitamin K, which is needed in the building of bone. Supplements of lactobacillus acidophilus and bifidobacteria bifidum can help replace this flora.
- Fluoride—When given in treatment doses, fluoride causes an apparent increase in bone mass, but the resulting bone is abnormal and lacks strength. Even small amounts of fluoride in common drinking water increases the risk of hip fracture.
- Insufficient calcium absorption—Calcium is ingested in the form of relatively insoluble salts, whether the source is food or supplements. To be absorbed, calcium requires not only vitamin D but adequate hydrochloric acid in the stomach. As we age, the amount of HCL secreted in the digestive system decreases. Since 50% of those 70 or older produce less HCL than is needed for calcium absorption, it would be prudent for them to take with meals a supplement of either HCL or calcium citrate, which is better absorbed under these conditions than other calcium compounds.

The best way to detect osteoporosis is by evaluating bone densitometry measurements. With the older concept of using x-rays for detection, one would have to have lost 30-40% of their bone mass before it would show up on the x-ray.

Osteoporosis is more common in aging women than heart disease, cancer, or Alzheimer's, affecting over 20 million American women at the close of this century. If one looks at the annual incidence of the following diseases, it is clear to see the impact of osteoporosis upon our senior years.

Fractures due to osteoporosis	1.3 million
Heart attack	513,000
Breast cancer	182,000

Uterine cancer	32,000
Ovarian cancer	26,000

I am sure many of you know someone who had a fracture, was admitted to the hospital, had successful surgery for the fracture, and then died due to complications from infections like pneumonia or blood clots to the brain or heart.

Treatments necessary for bone health include supplemental calcium, vitamin D, boron, progesterone, a weekly schedule of weight-bearing exercises, such as illustrated in *Chapter Three*, and if menopausal, HRT. Fosamax, a prescription drug released about two years ago, can also be a good adjunctive therapy for osteoporosis because it helps lay down new bone formation.

Our source of calcium can come from our diet, especially milk, broccoli, sardines, oysters, and spinach; however, in most cases, in order to receive the recommended daily dosage of 800 to 1500 mg it is necessary to take calcium supplements.

Obtaining adequate vitamin D can also pose an interesting problem, because in the absence of vitamin D, only 10% of calcium is absorbed. Milk, which many people consider a good source of vitamin D, is not always reliable, because numerous analyses of various milk companies have not revealed consistent quantities of vitamin D. Despite current UV phobia, sunlight promotes vitamin D. If you live in areas of the country like Vermont, the limited sunlight from November through March also decreases vitamin D production. Today, we have learned the usefulness of sunscreen creams to protect against the ultraviolet rays of the sun. The downside of this protection is that lack of sunshine markedly decreases vitamin D production. So, along with calcium, we need to take vitamin D supplements, 300 to 400 IU daily, and, if possible, welcome moderate sun exposure, unless you have a predisposition to skin cancer. As Frank comments in *Chapter Three*, nothing but fungus grows without sunshine. Just don't overdo it.

Boron, an important mineral for our bone health, potentiates estrogen's role in building bones and also helps conversion of vitamin D to the active form necessary for calcium absorption. Recommended dosage is usually about 3 mg daily. Taken with your calcium, preferably just before retiring, it promotes restful sleep.

HRT, as discussed earlier in the book, is very important in menopausal women and older men for good bone health.

Exercise, as we all know, is extremely important in our *Rage Against Age*. We all need to exercise regularly, but to assure good bone health, we must do weight-resistance exercises in order to maintain and increase our bone density. Frank has the bone density of a man half his age.

Viagra

Viagra was the first oral therapy for impotence, released by Pfizer in April of 1998. About 30 million men have erectile dysfunction, yet fewer than 10% have dared to come forward to ask for help because of embarrassment. Obviously, as we teach people to live longer and healthier, the question of the "Big One" (sexual impotence) will become more common, and hopefully, be more actively discussed by doctors with their patients, now that a simple, safe treatment is available.

The cyclic mechanism of erection of the penis involves release of nitric oxide in the corpus cavernosum, or spongy part of the penis, during sexual stimulation. The nitric oxide activates an enzyme, guanylate cyclase, which results in increased levels of cyclic quanosine monophosphate (cGMP), producing smooth muscle relaxation in the corpus cavernosum with subsequent inflow of blood. Viagra has no direct relaxant effect on isolated human corpus cavernosum, but enhances the effect of nitric oxide by inhibiting phosphodiesterase type 5, which is responsible for degradation of the cGMP in the corpus cavernosum. Sexual stimulation causes local release of nitric oxide. Viagra is unique in that it enhances an erection when a man is aroused, but has little to no effect in the absence of sexual stimulation. Viagra is effective in about 70% of men with sexual dysfunction from physical or psychological causes.

A thorough medical history and physical exam should be undertaken to diagnose erectile dysfunction, to determine potential underlying causes and before beginning appropriate treatment. There is an elevated degree of cardiac risk associated with more and vigorous sexual activity, especially among seniors, so physicians should consider the cardiovascular status of their patients, prior to initiating any treatment for erectile dysfunction. Viagra should not be taken by any patients using organic nitrates for angina or an elevated blood pressure condition. This combination has an additive hypotensive effect and may cause cardiac risk or syncope.

Viagra is available in three doses; 25 mg, 50 mg, and 100 mg. The starting dose for most men is 50 mg taken an hour before sex. In men over the age of 65 or those with severe kidney or liver impairment, the recommended starting dose is 25 mg. Also, the lower dose should be used for men taking the antibiotic erythromycin or anti-fungal medications like ketoconazole, as these drugs inhibit the metabolism of Viagra, because they all go through the same hepatic enzyme system - cytochrome P450. If after using the 50 mg dose on two or three occasions without reasonable results and there are no contraindications as outlined above, men can go to 100 mg, but they should discuss this option with their physician. In any event, Viagra should be limited to once daily dose. The effect of Viagra usually lasts from one to four hours. The most common side effects are minor headache, facial flushing, nasal congestion and indigestion, and an exhausted but gratified mate. These effects are transient, usually lasting up to three or four hours, Occasionally, some men (about 3%) will experience a temporary vision disturbance that makes it difficult to distinguish between the colors blue and green, but the impairment does not affect visual acuity. (Just don't make love to Martians!) This difficulty is due to the fact that in the retina of the eye there exists an enzyme called phosphodiesterase 6, similar chemically to the enzyme phosphodiesterase 5, which Viagra inhibits, as we discussed earlier.

Overall, Viagra has been quite successful in treating erectile dysfunction. Presently, continued research is being done on men as well as women, and probably in the not-too-distant future, there will be FDA approval of a similar medication for women as well. Before giving in to the life sentence of Viagra or celibacy, however, we strongly recommend an effort to boost your natural testosterone with DHEA, androstenedione, and Tribulus Terrestris (along with the prostate protectors Pygeum and Saw Palmetto). If you see no results in a month, consider physician-prescribed shots of testosterone cypionate. These supplements may not only match the effectiveness of Viagra, but may also give you the strength and endurance of a much younger man for a much longer period of time. Reach for the pleasure of a moment or the fuel for years of pleasurable experiences. Your choice.

Chapter Three

How to Combat Physical Deterioration

We are probably most conscious of the status of our bodies during the summer; it can be a distressingly embarrassing, brutally revealing season, The fancy clothes that have hidden us during the cooler months have become heavy and claustrophobic. The sun and the beach beckon. Mountain streams invite us to strip. Sheepishly, we suck in our guts and pull up our shoulders, as we look around the beach and peruse other aberrations of the human form. We find comfort in spying others of our vintage whose bodies have been misshapen by poor nutrition and lack of exercise, and we write off our own debilitation as a natural phenomenon of the aging process. Some of us look forward to the distant vacation, where we can peel off our clothes and not be ashamed of our decaying shapes, because no one there knows us. Others, too depressed with what poor habits have done to their bodies, will hide indoors during the long hot summer and rationalize their confinement with idiotic proclamations like, "avoid the sun, it's bad for your skin." (Have you ever tried to grow anything besides mold and fungi without sun?) Many people whose bodies have become grotesque from lack of use are blind to their self-destruction and think nothing of waddling beside the seashore in their size 50 bathing suits, guzzling one fattening beer or soft drink after another. Perhaps they rationalize that their peculiar shapes are predestined and uncontrollable. Perhaps they relate good physical conditioning to the realm of frivolous youth. It has been our observation that most people just do not think an athletic build is necessary: "Doesn't earn you any money" (the prime American motivator); "Doesn't attract women." (Some women are actually intimidated by well-developed bodies, probably because they are conscious of their own physical inadequacies, or perhaps they prefer to rationalize their mate's pathetic physical condition as "normal"); "It's not functional to have all that muscle." (Who needs it in today's industrialized society?) The excuses are familiar, but the fact remains: A well-tuned body, male or female, not only looks good, but will probably earn you active health and longevity if you maintain it properly.

Here again, we are misled by the popular notion that old age is far less than active and is not a particularly coveted state of being. Certainly, the majority of oldsters around us do not represent a necessarily happy lot. They are plagued with all kinds of degenerative illnesses and usually are dependent upon their nurses or young relatives for survival. *Time Magazine* in 1997 reported that a U.S. hospital survey revealed that one-third of their aged patients would rather die than be cared for in a nursing home, but the Centers for Disease Control's *Monthly Vital Statistics Report* of 1993 predicts that one of every two Americans living today will end up there. It does not have to be that way. For every ten men over 60 who are debilitated, there is one who is spry, self-dependent and productive. The body, like the mind, must be used if it is to remain alive, and that use should not stop at retirement. For some men, active use of the body stops as early as high school or college graduation. They comprise the thousands of early victims of cardiovascular and respiratory diseases. Richard A Passwater, in his brilliant book, *Super Nutrition* (1975), warned us: "Early indicators of the mortality rate predicted that the American median life span, which has been on a plateau for some twenty years, decreased between 1975 and 1985. This projected decrease had been blamed primarily on inactivity, smoking, suboptimal nutrition, and pollution of the air and water." At this closing of the 20th century, Passwater's observation has multiplied.

Industrialization has done a great deal to make our lives more comfortable; in the process, it has taken its toll on our health. All forms of mechanization and inventions for expediency and mass production have replaced man's muscular effort with his brain effort. Men take pride in not having to use their bodies. The laborer is looked down upon and even laughed at for not having the education or dollars that would advance him beyond the requirements of lowly manual effort. But the laborer, the farmer, the man who must use his body to earn a living, has the last laugh. He is living longer, a lot longer. And, he is not victimized by many of the ugly diseases that attack the non-laborer in his sunset years (that is, unless he smokes, consumes too much alcohol or commits nutritional suicide).

Man has survived the ravages of time because he had intelligence to do what was necessary for self-preservation, historically and prehistorically. But, that intelligence alone did not give him the strength to hunt or to run from those animals who hunted him. Only a well-conditioned body could meet those requirements. Before industrialization, man used his body to catch his staple foods, grow his vegetable and fruit supplements; he called upon his physical strength to hunt for the skins that covered his back, to transport himself and his family to new environments. In relation to all of recorded time, that was not too long ago. No process of mutation has lessened our capacity for these efforts. Automation has given man more comfort, but, together with the nutrition he has spoiled and adulterated by industrial processing, it has enfeebled man. Man has become a pathetic shadow of his powerful primitive self. Is it any wonder why, when today's "man" finds himself in an untimely primitive situation, like the physically demanding occasion of war, he finds himself physically inadequate and more inclined to cry, surrender or retreat?

The occasion that demands good physical conditioning need not be dramatic as war. How many men and women avoid exhilarating sports like skiing, simply because they cannot measure up to its adequate physical and courageous requirements? How many people would be of any good at all in an emergency situation where a little human power could save a life? We really should feel ashamed of ourselves for becoming a nation of pansies, more concerned with colognes, hair styles, and clothing than we are with our bodies, while dynamic women like Diana Nyad are challenging the ocean with heroic swims. But the primary reason for channeling some of those misdirected cosmetic concerns toward personal physical conditioning has nothing to do with heroic feats; it has a great deal to do with your capacity to achieve healthy active longevity. With a little effort, you can meet the debilitating aging process head on and put up a pretty good fight. The closer your body gets to the optimum silhouette that was its original design, the better chance you will have for a longer, active life. Dr. Robert Wiswell is an informed physician who believes in preventive maintenance. In an interview for *Modern Maturity* magazine, he admitted: "One thing I have observed is that for well-being, exercise is better than drugs. Activity combats atrophy."

The beacon that lights the way back to the natural mold has been before us for many years. We have been too busy trying to snuff out the light. We are talking about physical culture specifically as a result of training with weights. When the daily routine of our lives is devoid of survival challenges that would exercise our bodies, we must seek other forms of resistance to keep our bodies alive. While deprecating fools of this century have been laughing at men like Bernard McFadden, Eugene Sandow, Charles Atlas, Bob Hoffman, Jack LaLanne, Bill and Shawn Phillips, Mike Mentzer, and Joe Weider, the men responsible for true physical education in the U.S. and the sculpting of such magnificent forms as those displayed by the competitors of male physique contests, time has ironically put their critics in wheel chairs, sanitariums, and graves, while the followers of these inspiring physical culturists have led active lives well beyond what we consider to be old age. Some people can look at Ancient Greek and Roman statues of heroic men in all their muscular splendor and cry "art," when in the same breath they can look at their living counterparts in the flesh of bodybuilding champions like Arnold Schwarznegger (when he won the Mr. Olympia award) and put them down as muscle-bound "freaks." These deprecative comments usually come from men who are very soft or from women who are unnaturally hard.

We have heard the misinformed public accuse bodybuilders of every crime from egotism to sodomy, and wondered, why? For, in all of our 40 some odd years experience with men who pump iron, we have found most of them to be quite normal, different from their critics only in the respect that they are healthy specimens of woman and manhood, probably a lot closer in form to the original mold designed by our Creator. I have also never met one who was muscle-bound, another popular myth. Of course, the primary motivation for a man criticizing any other man is the pseudo-justification of his own inadequacy. "If what he's doing is wrong, then what I'm doing is right." Witness the overpowering influence of modern art. Our universities employ semanticist art professors who cannot paint like the Masters. They teach justification of "self-expressionism," and the gullible public has fallen for the hoax. Weak minds are led by what is fashionable. I will believe that Abstract Expressionism is not a hoax, when I find one modern "Master" who can paint as well as Bouguereau, taking the Abstract route by choice and not from technical inadequacy.

Some women refer to musculature as disgusting, odd, abnormal, weird. This observation helps them justify the soft, blubberous conditions of their husbands as normal. This ridiculing strategy is a familiar one in every walk of life, a defense to disguise our own inadequacies. Admittedly, some bodybuilders are on an incorrigible ego trip, but no more than are successful businessmen who take pride in how much more money and possessions they have than their neighbor. Most bodybuilders are into the sport only for self-improvement and the perpetuation of health. If ever tempted to boast of their progress, they have only to look at champions like Zane, Sergio Olivas, Schwarznegger, or Ron Coleman, and they will soon feel inferior.

You need not concern yourself with your potential to win physique contests. You can take part in the sport of bodybuilding without ever taking off your shirt. Self-improvement can be a private enterprise. The men who have won physique contests should serve as tangible examples of the ultimate in physical development. These men are quite real, have worked hard to attain their goal, and can teach us with authority. We have only to look, listen, and emulate. Take pride in not boasting of your progress, if that is your trip, but do train, because what these physical culturists are really peddling is a vital formula for health and active longevity at the nominal cost of just your participation. We have followed their methods, compared, analyzed, and applied their individual approaches. The results of our eclectic self-experiments are compiled in this book; in Frank's case, they represent over 50 years of such research and application. We have neither developed our bodies to Herculean proportions, nor do we aspire to win any contests, but we are a lot stronger, look a lot more symmetrical, and have a good deal more mental and physical energy than other men our age who have not benefited from good nutrition and sound progressive exercise. We expect to attain active health and longevity; these are our primary credentials for writing this book with authority. *Rage Against Age* is our personal testimony of effective diet, nutritional vitamins and supplements, and exercises of both body and mind which are helping us fight the debilitating, humiliating aging process.

If your doctor has warned you about weight-resistance exercise as being dangerous for those with high blood pressure, he has not kept up to date with his research. After 9 studies of 259 female and male subjects, researchers at Northern Illinois University of Dekalb concluded that weight training can reduce both systolic and diastolic blood pressure 3% to 5%, especially for those who already have a hypertensive condition.

Muscles and Myths

Although your bones may have stopped growing at about the age of 18, your muscle growth has no age limitation. The condition of your muscles right now is a result of environmental influences that either encouraged you to lead a physically active life or persuaded you to choose a life of lethargy. It is important for you to understand that the condition of your muscles has nothing to do with heredity. You may have inherited your bone structure, and that, of course, includes your height, but your bones are only the bare foundation of your total countenance, while your muscles and your fat create your silhouette. "But both my parents are fat," is frequently the excuse of the obese, who would like to place the blame of their shape upon heredity. What they really have inherited, besides their bone structure, is a lethargic life style that includes nonnutritious eating habits. But this latter type of inheritance is not genetic; it is behavioral. We have changed the shape of enough fat men and women to know that their physical condition has nothing to do with genetic inheritance. Frank Covino's present shape certainly is not inherited. His father was small, a lightweight. His mother was never over 100 pounds until she passed age 40. She, too, was short. Better nutrition made their children taller than their parents, but their three sons remained slight of build, ectomorphic. One of these skinny boys began to develop muscle and dense bone from progressive weight-resistance training and was able to transform his silhouette and increase his body weight by over 50 pounds in just two years. The newly acquired weight was mostly muscle. The newly acquired V-shaped silhouette was distinctly more masculine. The change brought about a self-confidence that affected his whole personality. From a withdrawn, inhibited, pathetically frail little boy with a fractured ego and a depressing inferiority complex, emerged a broad-shouldered young man, able to compete favorably with any other man, physically and mentally, in a new life of self-respect and significant achievement. Frank can testify that his present powerful physical stature has little to do with heredity. Moreover, his mental capacities would never have been expressed to the limit that he has used them, were it not for the ego-restoring change in his body. Any ectomorph can become a mesomorph with proper nutrition and weight-resistance exercise.

During his youth, Frank was also a victim of the team syndrome so characteristic of our culture. The "Little League" is a concept which, on the surface endeavors to teach our young boys how to cooperate with team effort, perhaps an admirable character developer for the boys who make "the team." But what about the boys who do not? What about the boys whose physical limitations make them of no value to the team effort? What about the boys "on the bench?" The effect should be obvious. Kids who cannot shape up to the expectations of "the team" feel the first taste of a butchered ego, and therein lies the basis of the inferiority complexes which follow them into adulthood. Team sports emphasis is thus a flagrant form of child abuse. Frank knows. He was one of the "kids on the bench." Moreover, his humiliation was compounded by the irony that his dad was the coach of the team. Team rejection drives a tortuous stake into the hearts of the rejected.

European and Asian schools are not team-oriented. Calisthenics and "individual development" activities which strengthen the body and the ego are more prevalent, particularly in the Communist bloc countries, which seem more bent on creating a society of poor but strong individuals, rather than a nation of rich, but physically sick capitalists. The business world of our nation is but an extension of the team syndrome, with corporations and their cooperative employees replacing the Little League. If an individual has nothing to offer the corporation, he does not "make the team." What has resulted is a nation of non-individuals, who have no identity beyond their use to their occupation. "What do you do?" is the opening question at every cocktail party, as if it is normal for a person to do just one thing, a totally unnatural phenomenon. Each of us has been gifted with far too much physical and mental potential for us to channel all our energies into one corporate direction. In the chapter regarding stress, we speak of separating the Self from roles we play in society, in an effort to realize as much of our individual physical and mental potentials as we can in one short lifetime. Such a reorganization of roles and sensible respect and protection of the Self is the only hope man has for leaving his personal mark upon the industrialized world. His alternative is to live in servile anonymity, and we question whether that is living at all.

Frank's father was a fantastic athlete. He was raised in a decrepit, poorly subsidized orphan home in Farmingdale, Long Island, where the food was less than meager and the nuns were more than strict. He had to battle for recognition by his peer group, since he was quite short. The fury of his fists became legendary. To keep the kids' minds off food the accent in "the home" was on physical activities, and all sports were offered. Frank's dad not only made every team, but was a star athlete. He left "the home" and become one third of a professional hand-balancing team which had a successful New York City Vaudeville run, before the Depression closed his curtain. In desperation, Frank Sr. entered the world of professional boxing, at which he did <u>very</u> well. He also started chain-smoking, fashionable in the Roaring Twenties. The cigarette became every tough guy's extremity. Taking a government job for "security," he married one of the girls on his mail route and promptly sired a son. Being the first born, Frank was expected to follow in his dad's athletic footsteps.

Unfortunately, Frank Jr. was a failure. At everything athletic. He ate poorly, and his lack of interest in physical activity kept him frail and small. Until high school, when he was first introduced to gymnastics and body building via progressive weight resistance. Without intending to kick sand in Charles Atlas' face, Frank exercised and gained an incredible 52 muscular pounds in one year. His new interest in muscle was accompanied by faster, denser bone growth, and he rapidly became more conscious of his <u>Self</u>. This self-awareness brought Frank into the fold. Psychologically, he recognized the agonizing team syndrome which had enfeebled him for ten years. Strength developed confidence, and his physical and mental achievements began to snowball. He had arrived, and he was so overwhelmed by his newly discovered capabilities that he went overboard to prove himself at a variety of sports activities. The curious thing is that they were not team-type sports; they included wrestling, boxing, gymnastics, rodeo riding, skiing, and surfing. He even took a shot at sky diving, before a miscalculation displaced his sacrum from his iliac. All this activity took place over two decades, punctuated by four years as a bewildered but fortunately effective soldier. We mention this, because the common denominator which permitted Frank to take part, and do fairly well, in these exciting activities, was his continued interest in body building with weights; from it, he gained strength, size, and self-discipline.

Although Frank's dad's physical pace was sufficient to dilate his arteries and decrease his resting heart rate to a healthy pulse, his poor early nutrition and heavy smoking habit eventually clogged his circulatory system, and the cumulative result, a fatal stoke, put him to his final rest before the age of 65. If he had known then what his son has learned since about nutrition and exercise, he might have been able to prolong his life. His untimely passing was a precious family loss, compounded by our opinion that it was totally unnecessary. We trust that the information we have provided in this book will prevent other such fatalities. If our book saves one life, our effort shall be well-expended.

This morning, a typical tourist family filed into the pew in front of ours at a small church in Miami Beach. The father had the two chins that commonly characterize a modern successful business man of 50 years. His wife had a derrière that spread three feet across, and her flesh spilled out of every opening in her bright red stretched Spandex clothing. Her child of nine had the same obese shape in a smaller form, and her son was also grossly overweight. Heredity? Studies have proven that what fat children really inherit from their parents is poor eating habits and lack of exercise. The refined sugar-and-starch-loaded breakfast the mother had just stuffed into her family that morning is another criminal form of child abuse. Children are totally dependent upon their parents for nutritional guidance. Any woman who deliberately makes of her children a carbon copy of her obese self has little respect for the privilege of motherhood. Any husband who permits such influence writes an early death warrant for himself and a life of misery and ridicule for his children. Given the option of losing the fat or blowing the marriage, most men and women would take better care of themselves. Make it easy for your mate by going on a joint self- improvement program. Involve your child, too. You will be proud of the health that your family radiates in a short time, and your children will "inherit" your new physically fit life style.

What we truly inherit is our bone structure, and, possibly, our rate of metabolism. The fat and muscle (or lack of it) around your bones was planted there by your closest environmental influences and then shaped by your own choice of life style. If exercise and good nutrition were parts of that life style, you have extended your years of life expectancy. If you chose the hedonistic, most popular, indolent route, you may have shortened that life span. Whether you ameliorate your present condition is another choice you will have to make, after reading this book.

Before beginning your exercise program, we would like to challenge a few myths and convenient rationalizations which have collectively influenced the life style of most contemporary men and women.

"Weight lifters are egotistic mesomorphs (muscular men) who have developed their bodies in lieu of their minds."

It has been our experience that many significant achievements by man had egoistic motivation. There is an important difference between egoism and egotism: The former is a personal strive for excellence, a primary concern for self-improvement, without which man would not come close to realizing his mental and physical potentials. Egotism is characteristic of the braggart, that is the repulsive conceit which most of us find intolerable; but, there are egotists involved in every activity. It is not an exclusive characteristic of the weight-lifting community. In fact, the greater percentage of those involved in body building is comprised of men who feel inferior, badly enough to work hard for the amelioration of their inadequate physical condition.

Mesomorphs develop easily and usually have experienced a sufficient amount of athletic successes during their youth to have developed a strong, shapely body without the assistance of weight training; the young men we refer to as natural athletes usually fall into this category. Whether they stay in that condition or not depends upon whether they continue their athletic involvement beyond graduation. If they totally discontinue physical activity, they are prime candidates for cardiovascular disease, despite their pre-developed muscular countenance. At any rate, mesomorphs surprisingly represent the smallest percentage of men who lift weights. They are the least likely to recognize its value and the most likely to put down the activity as one that is non-athletic, since it lacks the basic element of game type competition. Hit and conquer! Mesomorphs who become physically inactive after school graduation (high school or college) more often than not turn into endomorphic sports spectators, the fat-bellied beer guzzlers, whose derrières conceal their barstools. These TV football game watchers are generally the strongest voices heard against physical development through the use of weights, probably because the young personal body they remember "came naturally," and many of them are of the mistaken notion that you are either born with it or you are not.

Too many doctors and undergraduate students are involved in body building today, via progressive weight resistance, for any informed adult to believe the last part of this tired first myth any longer. The finest and most highly respected heart surgeons in the world recognize the cardiovascular benefits of progressive overload activities like weight training, and they believe in this form of exercise enough to engage in the lifting of weights themselves. Dr. Charles Anderson is one of them. Check with your own local cardiologist for corroboration of this widely indicative contemporary acceptance by health-conscious physicians. Body builders who train with weights are as well-educated today as any sportsmen and probably are more socially acceptable, since they are not dominated by the odious motivation of *conquest* in their physical activity. The atmosphere in a weight room is one of camaraderie and extreme individual effort in a common bond, directed toward one adversary, the debilitating aging process. The weight lifting gymnasium is a true fountain of vibrant youth, and, since they started admitting women, the gyms are a lot cleaner. They have replaced single bars for social contacts. Meet your mate there, and you are less likely to hook up with a loser.

"I've heard that you get fat when you stop exercising with weights."

Another myth usually fostered by those who are painfully thin or by those who just need an excuse for not participating. If an obese man would make the effort to change his shape by exercising with weights and adjusting his diet, he would in time succeed. If he then stopped and resumed his previously deleterious life style of no exercise and malnutrition, he would most certainly regain his obesity. It has been our observation that any man will revert back to his original pre-exercised condition, if he discontinues exercise and sensible nutrition. If Frank stops training for a prolonged length of time, he gets a lot thinner, reverting to his ectomorphic state that characterized him before he began to train with weights During the Korean War, his body weight dropped to 145 lbs. He tilts the scale today at 190, carrying less then 10% body fat. You have the capacity to sculpt any shape of body you desire, if you apply yourself to a regenerative routine; this indicates that your commitment to body building must be a change in life style that you will continue for the rest of your life. Would you make such a commitment? You have been given a marvelous machine in your Self that functions with a body and a mind, but you have to push the buttons. To let either part die, or atrophy in lethargy, is to contribute to the premature destruction of that machine, and you have no one to blame for that deterioration but yourself. Have you been unconsciously suicidal?

"I'm too out of shape. Lifting weights will give me a heart attack."

At least you recognize your poor condition. It is never too late to strengthen any muscle, and that includes the heart, unless there has been some damage to the brain. Sensible exercise which keeps your heart pulsing at about 75% of its maximum rate for short periods during one hour out of every other day will strengthen your heart and enlarge the diameter of your arteries, providing a proven defense against our nation's number-one killer, cardiovascular disease. Dr. Morris Crawford, writing for the British Medical Journal, stated that the increasing proclivity for coronary disease could be reduced significantly by engaging in heavy exercise, such as that which involves progressive weight resistance. Most physicians, recognizing the heart as a muscle, now prescribe mild exercise even for patients who are recovering from a heart attack. In his inspirational book, *The Jack LaLanne Way to Vibrant Good Health* (1960), Jack calls the heart "the most durable muscle in your entire body. It works for you from the start of your life to the end, hour in and hour out, by day and by night, in sickness, health, sadness or elation. It was made to work. Every exercise you perform strengthens the heart and no exercise, properly performed, will injure it." The correlation between cardiovascular deaths and lethargic life styles has been clearly supported by the Framingham study, as has the relationship between low physical activity and hypertension with elevated serum cholesterol been proven, especially among cigarette smokers, according to S.G. Haynes (1978).

<u>"I'm a businessman. I have no need for the strength and shape of a weight lifter. Jocks are abnormal."</u>

Israeli Dr. Daniel Brunner remarked to the American Heart Association that businessmen and sedentary workers are three times more susceptible to heart disease than are more physically active laborers. An international team of researchers, investigating the causes of atherosclerosis proved that the primary fault lies with physical <u>inactivity</u> In an address to the Chicago College of Physicians, Dr. Wilhelm Raab, a member of that research team, expressed alarm that doctors should refer to the athlete's larger heart and dilated arteries as stress induced abnormalities. "It's not the so-called 'athlete's heart' which should be considered abnormal," suggested the physician, "but rather the degenerating, inadequate 'loafer's heart' which should be dubbed abnormal."

Even a businessman should be prepared for exigencies that place him under severe mental and physical stress. In a report from a joint committee of the American Medical Association and the Association for Health, Physical Education and Recreation, we are cautioned that "in emergencies of various types, sudden and unusual physical demands may be laid upon individuals and groups. The possession of physical strength, agility and endurance may enable the individual or group to survive, while the lack of fitness may spell catastrophe." Make the fatal mistake of "spending your health to gain your wealth," and, one day, you will wake up rich but prematurely old, and all the money in the world cannot buy active longevity. The National Office of Vital Statistics lists coronary diseases and heart failures as responsible for over 900,000 deaths annually in this country. Can you afford to gamble with those figures? W. Bortz, in a 1980 article in the *Journal of the American Geriatric Society*, stated that exercise has proven to be an important key to conquering the aging process, and it can cost you nothing!

<u>"Lifting weights sounds too much like work. I would rather spend money on a fat reducing machine or ride a bicycle."</u>

In the May-June 1978 issue of *Consumers Digest* magazine, an anonymous author had these interesting words to say about exercise machines: "Ads showing Farrah Fawcett and other beautiful actresses swinging away at exercise machines are saying that you too can be a beautiful young actress if you enroll in some course or buy an expensive machine. But actresses are beautiful before they are given machines, and ads are simply another role they play—for money. Like most roles, the ads have the slenderest [very appropriate adjective] of relationships with reality. The divine Farrah didn't get that way from a machine. Neither will you. The machine might make a few shekels for its owner, but only a bicycle machine that you actually pump with the same effort it takes to ride the real thing will be of any benefit to you."

We could not be more in agreement, and this entire article would have taken its place in our morgue of brilliant prose were it not for a bit of uninformed reporting it also included: The phantom author later deprecates, "weight lifting, barbells, and other paraphernalia of muscle building," as having nothing to do with health, "and they can also be dangerous." Someone should enlighten that writer, [no doubt, a pencil-neck] who may not realize that the heart is one of those vital muscles which certainly can be developed with an overload program of progressive weight-resistance exercise. He should also be informed that the development of any muscle will be the development of an auxiliary heart which will help transport the blood more efficiently through the circulatory system. A contracted muscle pushes blood toward the heart and when the muscle relaxes, it draws blood away from the heart to engorge itself. This flush action is exactly what the heart does. The danger that may challenge the weight lifter is mild (at worst, a strained or severely torn muscle) when compared to the danger of leading a sedentary life devoid of exercise, which surely will result in premature aging and early mortality. Strained muscles are almost always the result of strenuous exercise that is not preceded by a related light warm-up. Educated weight lifters are well aware of this precaution and seldom sustain injury. The only other weight-lifting danger we can imagine is a broken toe, from dropping a plate on it. We have never seen this happen, but the probability of such an accident has increased, as the workout clothing for women has become briefer, and the testosterone levels of weight lifters has increased. Of course, it would be foolish for anyone with a known poor heart condition to begin a heavy strenuous weight-lifting program. Your participation should be related to your personal heart condition, revealed by measuring its pulse at rest and under exertion. We will teach you how to measure your pulse, how to apply it, and how to ameliorate it with the exercise program in this book. But no one should begin any exercise routine until you have had a complete physical and discussed the program with your doctor. It is assumed that you will select a doctor who is an excellent example of health and fitness himself.

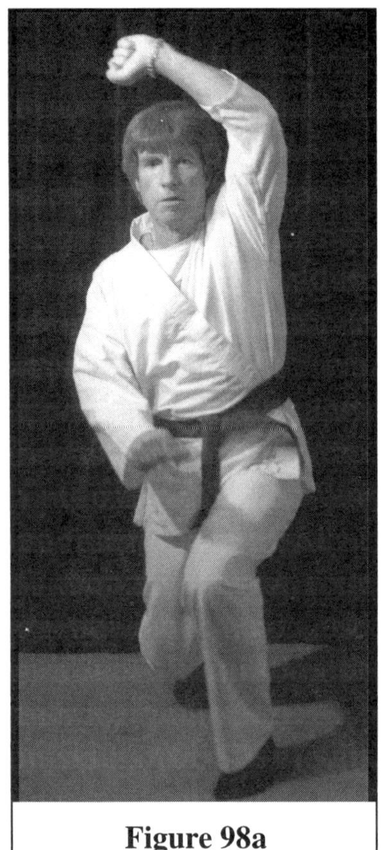

Figure 98a

Dr. Charles Anderson, Brown Belt

The act of pressing down on a bicycle pedal is no different from pushing away a weight with the same leg. The weight provides the same type of resistance as does the revolution of the bicycle wheel, but pushing weights with the leg, or legs, has the added advantage of being stress-controllable. In addition, a weight-lifting program designed for your entire body will improve your posture. Bicycle pedaling is an exhilarating sport, and you certainly should consider cross-training as a supplement to your bodybuilding program, but to choose it as your only form of exercise is asking for no more physical development than the muscular conditioning of your legs, entirely dependent upon how much you use your high gears. Bicycling up hill is a good form of resistance exercising. Cross-training with sports like karate (Fig. 98a) and downhill skiing (Fig. 99b) will make your muscles functional and sharpen your reflexes, but progressive weight-resistance exercise will develop the strength you need to perform well at these other activities.

Your cardiovascular system can be ameliorated only if your activity is constant for 30 minutes, interrupted by intervals of extreme exertion. The amount of resistance must be increased periodically or the exercise will have no ameliorative value. On the bike, this means welcoming periods of challenge, like riding uphill. In the weight room, the weight resistance must be increased to provide stress, once the muscles involved cease to exert maximum effort after a specified number of repetitions. These increases of resistance are what physical culturists refer to as "progressive overload." If the strenuous efforts are bridged with intervals of lesser efforts instead of rests, you will be dispersing lactic acid which stiffens the muscles that have been stressed, and you will be training your cardiovascular system at the same time. These lesser effort intervals are represented by the flat runs while bicycling (if the cyclist continues to pedal rather than coast) and by periods of what Dr. Laurence Morehouse calls "active rest" between sets of weight-lifting exercises.

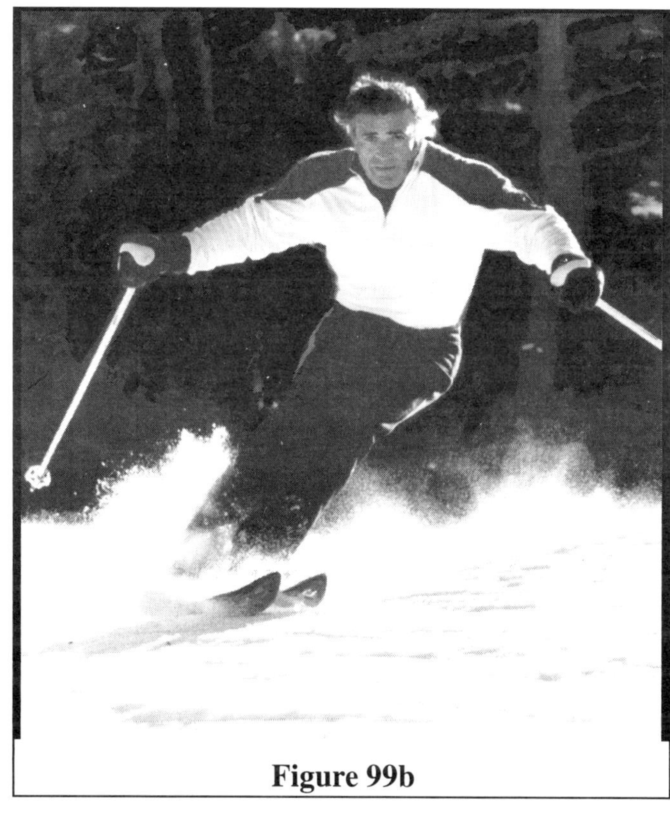

Figure 99b

Frank Covino, 67, Professional Skier

If the weight lifter rests completely and for too long between exercises, he will lose the ameliorative cardiovascular value of his efforts. His "pumped" muscles might grow, but the efficient flow of his blood would not necessarily improve, and his endurance might be hindered. Strong muscles alone will not stretch your lifespan, but an efficient cardiovascular system, marked by a low resting heart rate <u>will</u> certainly prolong the aging process. This is achieved by enlarging the diameter of your arteries, a condition that is sure to follow any sustained exercise program that includes progressive overload and interval training. Dr. Morehouse believes that "only with circulorespiratory development do you have a program that will serve all your needs," in his 1975 book, *Total Fitness in Thirty Minutes a Week.*

Dr. Morehouse's incredibly short exercise program, though, begs the pertinent question: "Fit for what?" His contention is that modern living places no demands upon man to require the body of a Mr. America. His principal effort is to improve your cardiovascular system to a minimum level for good health. A bare minimum. Our program promises health plus strength and youthful musculature through your senior years. Though we personally believe that the benefit you will derive from Dr. Morehouse's gentle, limited exercise program is minimal (unless you are in really bad condition), his theories directed toward an improvement of your cardiovascular system are sound, making his book a vital addition to your health library. He is pampering his readers, though, who, we are certain, welcome the idea that they can become "fit" by applying no more than ten minutes of effort three times a week; that sells books. We have learned that there are no short cuts to total physical development; no ten-minute plans that will effect dramatic changes. Your body was meant to work, hard enough to battle and hunt prehistoric animals. If you think you can develop it beyond its most basic potential by coddling yourself with ten-minute programs that promise quick results, you are either pitifully naive or you are kidding yourself. Be a pragmatist. Test any program you read for credibility. Choose the program that has most obviously contributed to your health and your physical stature. No one can judge better than yourself.

"I've got a bad back: hurt it playing football in college. I can't lift weights."

Pat Matson, who spent ten years as an offensive guard in the National Football League with the Denver Broncos, the Cincinnati Bengals, and the Green Bay Packers, suffered eight injuries which required major surgery. Twenty years ago he opened a physical fitness center in Cincinnati, where he has helped rehabilitate many other injured athletes. Pat had this to say to Barry Sparks, in an interview for *Strength and Health Magazine*: "One of the most effective tools a person can employ in order to recover from an injury is weight lifting. Not only will it allow the athlete to isolate certain body parts on which he wants to concentrate, but he will be able to control the amount of resistance involved. In addition, it builds strength, increases range of motion, promotes endurance, and decreases an athlete's chance of injury."

You should know that the science of bodybuilding differs from the science of weight lifting; the former provides formulas for spot development of body parts for people who want to sculpt their bodies into a particular shape, while the sport of weight lifting provides formulas for hoisting great poundages overhead with a singular exerted effort. This book is a primer that will provide some of those body sculpting formulas for you. If you have incurred an injury of any sort, it is certainly possible for you to strengthen the muscles around that wound and most probably, with time, negate its debilitating influence.

Several years ago, Frank sustained an injury from a bad landing while sport parachuting. It was a frustrating experience because I could not pin the blame for my demise upon any miscalculation. After a perfect exit from the plane, I opened my chute for a gentle float down from 2500 feet. It was a clear day and the sky was all mine, as I looked up to see the transport climb to a higher altitude for the more experienced sky divers. Slowly, I pulled down on the left toggle to steer toward the target area. The chute's gore functioned on cue. The steering was dead accurate. Suddenly, at about 500 feet, I heard this voice, loud and clear: "Right turn! Right turn!" It had to be God, I thought; no one else was up there. Then again, "Right turn," one of the Jumpmasters was bleating through a loudspeaker on the ground. "Right turn?" But there was a lake to my right, and the target area was to my left. Also, the wind was coming from my left, unless somebody starched the windsock at the tower. I continued steering into the wind, certain that the Jumpmaster was mistaken. Then it hit. One of those turbulent ground winds that swirl like a hurricane. I could not see it from my elevation, but on the ground it clearly cut a swath of spinning sand across the landing field. It caught me at about 100 feet and I plummeted. Instinctively, I looked down and retracted my legs, when the ground rushed toward me. One of the first lessons in sky diving is to never look down during the last part of your descent. The second lesson is never retract your legs. An almost straight body will absorb the landing shock and facilitate your parachute landing fall (PLF). Scrunched up in a fetal position, I hit the dust like a shell from a Howitzer and literally dug a crater in the ground.

A fractured ankle, two torn meniscus pads, and a subluxation of my iliac, which still pops out at least once every ski season, topped the list of injuries. The hip injury was a painful one, which three orthopedic doctors agreed would never allow me to ski again. I could have accepted that sentence, as many athletes have, and slowly sunk into a life of self-pity and indolence, as the fat accumulated around my bones. Instead, I opted for hyper-development of the muscles around the injured areas by following a program of progressive weight-resistance exercises specifically designed for that part of my body. I had been away from body building for several years, and it felt good to get back into it. As long as I had to be in the gym to cure my condition, I reasoned, I might as well throw in a few other exercises and see if my body would still respond at the late age of "pushing forty." The body did respond, and I was skiing better than ever two seasons later. Since then, I have continued to tone the muscles of my body with progressive weight-resistance exercises during at least three seasons of the year. Downhill skiing is the only form of exercise I need in the winter, an excellent anaerobic and cardiovascular training. Unlike most other sports, snow skiing exercises just about every muscle in the body, with particular emphasis upon the legs and abdomen. If I must relegate that exercise to just the few days of the weekend, I will push weights during the week. My wife Barbara is a supportive workout partner. She skis with the grace of an eagle.

Strength is a natural long lasting high. It is a very secure, comfortable feeling to know that your body is ready for any physical challenge. A strong body could save your life, or the life of somebody else, and it is never too late to strengthen any part of your body, unless you have damaged your central nervous system. As we mentioned earlier in this book, you are totally in control of your own destiny, but if that future is to be characterized by active longevity, you must use your body and all that requires is a brain.

We have discussed myths and popular rationalizations that keep many people from conditioning their bodies with weights. There are more, enough to fill a book, and each excuse can be blown apart with truthful contradictory testimony. We will not consider any others now, as there is more important work ahead. Let us begin by examining your pulse, so that the program you select will be directed toward your own physical condition. If you have not done anything physical for 20 years, you are not expected to follow an exercise program designed for the massive Dorian Yates (former Mr. Olympia), although the exercises could be the same. What would differ is the quantity of weight resistance and the frequency of the lifts. As a matter of fact, the course designed by Morehouse is an excellent one for anyone who has not engaged in physical activity for a long time. The course's only flaw is that it does not provide an exercise for the development of every principal muscular area; that would take more than ten minutes three days out of the week. We are concerned with total muscular development along with the maintenance of an efficient cardiovascular system. The ten minutes per alternate day plan will get you longevity; our plan will deliver active longevity with a youthful muscular body even into your sunset years. You alone can modify the manifestations of the aging process.

We should mention that our knowledge of cardiovascular amelioration monitored by pulse rate is a theory totally influenced by the book we have mentioned and Morehouses's 1977 excellent second book, *Maximum Performance*. In compiling our extemporization, we tested dozens of physical culturists theories and diets, in order to give this book eclectic credence. No information passed on to you has been taken for granted, as we are fully aware that too many individuals are influenced by whatever they read, under the mistaken notion that whatever is in print must be truthful. We offer photos as empirical evidence of our considered conjecture. It is assumed and certainly recommended that you take part in no exercise or nutritional program before taking a complete physical and discussing your participation in the self-improvement routine with a qualified medical practitioner.

The Heart Rate

The pulse is a good barometer, as it measures the beat of the heart against the blood in your circulatory system. Its count can indicate your emotional status, your body temperature, your muscular effort, and the efficiency of your circulatory blood flow. The term maximal heart rate relates closely to maximal oxygen consumption and can be used to measure that efficiency. We are particularly interested in measuring your pulse rate when you are at rest and also when you are involved in physical effort of moderate to heavy intensity. These measurements are what is known as your heart rate. Tests have indicated that low resting heart rates, pulsing at below 65 beats per minute are generally indicative of good health, particularly if the subject's pulse rate returns to that low rate soon after completing a bout of exercise that pushed the pulse up beyond a moderate effort rate of 120. The heart rates of professional athletes involved in sports which tax the cardiovascular system have been measured as low as 50 pulse beats per minute in their resting state. After a 12-month cardiovascular training program, I was able to lower my own resting pulse rate from 72, which is about "normal," to 64, primarily from exercising with weights and by using the progressive overload and interval training system. It may interest you to know that this lowering was accomplished after reaching the age of 60. Though I had trained on and off with weights since high school days, my former efforts were directed toward muscular development alone. It is only during the past few years that these efforts were also directed toward cardiovascular improvement. Muscular development was an additional benefit. You may be shocked, as we were, to learn that you can actually train your cardiovascular system and improve it while developing your muscular form.

Doctors and nurses traditionally find the pulse of their patients by gently pressing their middle fingertip upon the radial artery under the wrist at the base of the thumb. You can also measure your pulse by finding the carotid artery just before the sternocleidomastoid muscle under the jaw (Fig. 104a). Medics count the pulse beats for an entire minute. For our purposes, when measuring the heart rate after exercise, it would be better to measure the number of pulse beats in six seconds and multiply by ten, as six seconds is a good deal closer to the moment of your peak exertion than is 60, and the reading for a full minute would not be as accurate. Keep your eye on the second hand of a clock; when it reaches one of the five-minute marks, say the word zero. Then begin your count at the first beat beyond the starting point. Measure your resting heart rate right now, while you are reading this book. It may take a few tries before you find your pulse. Your beating pulse will be lowest after a good night's sleep and can be as much as ten beats per minute higher just before you retire. For a mean reading, measure it midday, and not too close to just after mealtime, as the metabolic conversion of ingested calories can elevate your reading.

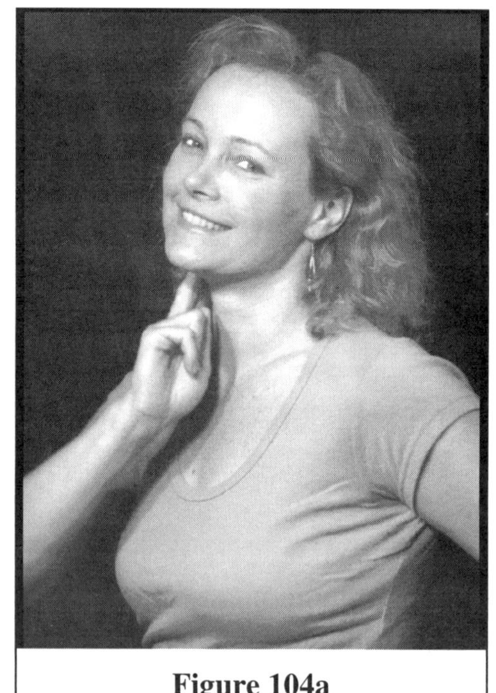

Figure 104a

Barbara Covino measures her pulse at the carotid artery just under the jaw.

We have mentioned that an optimum pulse for cardiovascular training during your exercise period would be about 75% of whatever your maximum heart rate is. You can find out your maximum heart rate by submitting to a stress test offered by a qualified cardiologist. A simpler, roughly accurate method has been recommended by Morehouse and is valid for anyone who has not already been finely tuned and accustomed to heavy exercise. He advises that you subtract your age from the number 220 for an approximation of your maximum heart rate and multiply that by the percent of maximum effort you chose to exert for your training pulse rate. Thus, 220 minus your age (say 40) would be 180; multiply by 75% and you get a training pulse rate of 135 (75% of maximum effort pulse) for a 40-year-old. Experienced athletes can safely bump that percentage to 85%. Weight training with high intensity can soar it even higher.

Morehouse has proven that the cardiovascular system can be trained effectively by subjecting yourself to exercise that keeps your pulse elevated between 60% and 80% of your maximum level for "compact" periods of only ten minutes during three days a week, with a rest day following each training day and a long rested weekend. Mild exercise such as walking would be sufficient if you are obese or in very poor physical condition. Dr. Art Mollen, in his book titled, *Future Youth*, agrees that ten minutes is a good beginner's goal "because that's the minimum addictive dose." Once you get hooked, go for 30 minutes, then an hour. By thc time one hour feels perfunctory, you will be ready for weight-resistance exercise.

Experimenting upon himself, Frank has effected the most rapid muscular development and cardiovascular amelioration (indicated by muscle size and a progressively lowered resting heart rate) by following a four-day-per-week schedule of weight-resistance bodybuilding exercises for about a 60-minute period; this schedule is stressful enough to push his active heart ratc to between 80% and 90% percent of maximum effort. The calibration is as follows: 220 minus his age of 67 = 153, multiplied by .85 = 130.05, or a training pulse of about 130 beats per minute during each set of the exercise period (which generally lasts about one hour). Active rest periods of no longer than one minute follow every ten-minute "compact" set of his exercises, performed at 80% to 90% of his maximum heart rate. He allowed longer rest periods between sets of exercises designed for different parts of his body.

When he tried the same program daily, allowing only Sunday as a day of rest and restricting his diet to mostly protein with limited carbohydrates and fats, he lost thirteen pounds and became hard as a rock, but Frank was thoroughly exhausted. We have concluded that such a daily routine is effective for younger men. The body needs a fair chance to recuperate from stressful activity, and we believe that need expands with age. A one-hour bout of exercise three or four days a week, working a different body part each session, seems to be an ideal program. Such a program is beneficial for most men <u>and women</u>. To avoid injury, it is also advisable to stretch and warm-up with light sets of high repetitions of each exercise, before concentrated effort using heavier weights.

"I like to lower the repetitions, as I increase the weight resistance," adds Frank, "Muscular development can only occur if you work to failure; the last repetition of each exercise should be really difficult. Advanced body builders often complete their sets with a more rapid aerobic set of low weight and 100 repetitions. The weight should be heavy enough to make the one hundredth repetition very difficult. This is a great way to include cardiovascular training with anaerobic exercise. You will be amazed at the strength and energy that ensues."

The great thing about using the heart rate as a measure of your progress is that it is as individual as your fingerprint, and is far more meaningful with regard to your longevity than is your strength or the size of your muscles. Most bodybuilding programs list a series of exercises and advise the participant to lift until he cannot, and, when it gets too easy for a specified number of repetitions, add more weight. This series surely will develop muscle, but we reach farther. Our cardiovascular approach to bodybuilding is as concerned with internal development as it is with strength and external appearance. It follows a similar system of progressive overload as most body building systems prescribe, but it advises the beginning participant to lift until his heart rate climbs about 60% of the person's maximum; then, to <u>keep it there</u> for however long it takes to complete the set of exercise; then to lower it to about 50% of maximum while "actively" resting, then go on to another exercise, again taxing the heart at 60% of maximum effort. A more extensive rest period may take place between the exercise of different parts of the body. These longer recuperative periods are especially important for men over 40, but should never exceed three minutes.

Advanced bodybuilders work out at over 90% of their maximum effort; their hearts are strong enough to bear such a load. Beginners who are really out of shape should not exert themselves above 60% of their maximum effort. The heart is a muscle that can be trained, but can also be strained. A good training pulse rate for men who have not gone entirely to pot and who might take part in other sports is 75%. Four weeks are a good spread for heart adjustment; i.e., begin working out at 60% of 220 minus your age and stay at that level for four weeks. Progressively increase your pulse during exercise by 5% every 4 weeks. By the 24th week, you will be lifting at 90% of your maximum effort, and that is about the limit, unless you are a champion.

Dr. Jan Karlsson was one of a group of Swedish physiologists who made a comprehensive study of the amount of physical effort, measured by the heart rate, expended by two 25-year-old Alpine skiing champions. It was reported in *Skiing Magazine* that during 45 minutes of slalom training, their average heart rates varied from 100 to 205 beats per minute, with the low calibration taken while the skiers were on the lift and the incredibly high calibration taken during giant slalom competitions of approximately 95 seconds. That rate is curiously well beyond maximum effort, as the maximum heart rate of the skiers was determined to be no higher than 199 prior to the experiment. This discrepancy can be explained by the fact that an athlete in competition experiences mental stress with its resulting adrenal secretions which, in turn, compound the stress of muscular challenge and raise the heart rate to incredible heights. Physiologists refer to this phenomenon as the stress adaptation syndrome, a phrase borrowed from Dr. Hans Selye. Professional bodybuilders lift weights to the point of physical failure, and their followers are advised to do the same in order to realize maximum muscular development, but that failure is largely dependent upon their pain quotient, their testosterone level, and upon their real determination to reach their goal. Many are consciously or subconsciously willing to achieve less that the massive perfection of Mr. Olympia, and their heart rates during exercise reflect that satisfaction with mediocrity. "No gain without pain" is a well-known phrase quipped in many gymnasiums. The choice is yours. Settle for painless mediocrity or tolerate the natural pain of muscular stress and "go for the gold." It's attainable—especially when natural hormones like nandrolone or peaked testosterone are your octane. We have recommended precursors that are available for you over the counter.

Using the 75% to 80% of maximum heart rate as an average training pulse guide, readers should regulate the intensity of their workout to a stress that demands about 150 pulse beats per minutes during each set of exercise, if they are between the ages of 25 and 35. A set is usually comprised of 8 to 10 repetitions of a specific exercise. Those between 35 and 45 should work out at about 140 pulse beats per minute. Those between 45 and 55 should try for a training pulse rate of about 130. Those over 55 would be wise to go lower yet, unless they are in top physical condition. Remember, these are average rates, which means you would be wise to begin lower and increase 5% every four weeks, as we have advised. As your muscles develop, your own heart will signal that it is capable of increased effort. With weight training, that means either increasing the quantity of repetitions or increasing the poundage. More repetitions during each exercise will result in greater muscular definition (particularly if coupled with a low carbohydrate and saturated fat, high-protein diet). Added weight resistance will increase muscular size and strength, particularly if the negative or eccentric part of the movement (return from full muscular contraction) is done slowly. Slow negatives place a lot of stress upon the joints, though. Many bodybuilders guard against this stress by taking supplement tablets of MSM, Chondroitin Sulphate and Glucosamine Sulphate, along with Phosphatidyl Serine, a proven defense against the stress hormone cortisol, which can actually be catabolic. Frank takes 400 mg of Phosphatidyl Serine daily for protection against this form of muscle wasting. Catabolism, a form of sell-cannibalism, can also be guarded against by daily ingestion of a minimum of one gram of protein for every pound of body weight, once you begin your body building program, with the greatest amount of calories eaten shortly after your workout. You have about a two-hour window to renourish the muscles you have stressed, before cortisol begins its catabolic attack. A meal that includes at least 40 grams of protein, 150 grams of complex carbohydrates, 5 grams of creatine, and 2 grams of glutamine is recommended at this time, unless you are deliberately on a ketogenic diet to lose fat. For fat depletion and muscular definition, cut the carbs down to no more than 15 grams and keep protein at 40 grams. You will have to skip the creatine, though, as it demands carbohydrate for insulin transport. Fats should never exceed 40 grams for daily consumption, and should preferably be of the unsaturated types, with flaxseed oil and fish oils heading the preferential list.

Developing Muscle for Powerful Longevity

"Live fast. Die young, and have a good looking corpse!" is a memorable line from an old paperback novel that teenagers have come to adopt as their credo, during the late years of the 20th century. Cults covet credos; they inspire passion and cult unity. Unity of any mass group gives its members power. Many adults fear teen power. So much of the strength felt by youth is based upon the frailty they witness in the aged. "They are weak. We are strong!" It is part of the most basic "survival of the fittest" syndrome. The lyrics of their popular music have provided subliminal mortar for the wall that separates most teens from the rest of society. Anger and recalcitrance mark their flag. They trample the weak and ridicule the aged.

Let us focus upon their puzzling desire to "die young." Why do teens find senior years so undesirable? Why does the milestone of 30 appear as a gravestone to our youth? There is little wonder that a teenager would embrace the suicidal drop-out credo, when its alternative, "Live gently. Die old, and have a fat repulsive corpse, crippled for years with osteoporosis, obesity, diabetes or cancer, kidney failure, and all the other debilitating diseases that characterize the aged," paints a frightening, certainly undesirable, image. Why would anyone want to face that terrifying sentence? I was raised to believe in the "resurrection of the body" after death. Which body, I continue to wonder, the body that you had at 18…25? Certainly you would not want it to be the decrepit body you see on some people at age 40, 50 or 70. Take a walk through any shopping mall. Which body would you bring to heaven, then? The truth is that your Creator has given you the potential for development of a beautiful body. You could look like an ancient Greek or Roman statue, but He has also given you a free will to develop that body or to <u>choose to let it waste</u>. Which path do you think is more sinful? The aged body that teenagers reject when they opt to "live fast" and "die young" is an aberration of what the Lord intended, a debilitated state that has resulted from <u>neglect</u>, from <u>lethargy</u>, and from the seemingly ubiquitous sin of <u>gluttony</u>. One look at the powerful, though aged, Leonardo, well into his senior years, painted by Raphael in his "School of Athens," as a model for Plato, indicates that man did not always have disrespect for his body. Renaissance men tried to emulate the men of Plato's era, where the goal was perfection of the mind, body and spirit. Those men were powerful but the Industrial Revolution changed that. We live in a utilitarian society where our primary physical and mental energies are directed toward one common goal: self-gratification from little physical effort.

Western civilization has bred legions of lethargic hedonists who lose about 5% of their muscle every ten years after they hit the age of 30. The type of muscle most frequently lost is called fast twitch fiber, and its loss is <u>totally from lack of use</u> against formidable resistance, like the charge of a dinosaur or the weight of a boulder that can block the entrance to your cave from predators; it is the type of muscle you presently need to be able to lift your luggage. There is a great wisdom in the cliché, "Use it or lose it!" Every time I hear thunder, I imagine the Creator bellowing to the latest arriving group of "resurrected" bodies: "I gave you the capacity to develop a body as beautiful as a Phidias marble, and you bring me this?" Look in the mirror. Naked. How close have you come to developing your potential?

It truly does not have to be that way. You could "Live active. Die old, but strong, and have a great looking corpse," and your self-improvement program can begin at any age. Youth is not a pre-requisite of physical attractiveness. Give your teenage grandchildren something to look forward to. Seniors, would you want to look like you, if you were a teen? Some of you may feel exonerated for writing off appearance as an egotistical, frivolous pursuit, but a strong body will create a more efficient cardiovascular system to nourish your heart and stimulate your brain. A rejuvenated brain will make you more aware, and hopefully, more productive, thereby justifying your existence. Intellectual productivity will elevate you above the level of animals, who are quite capable of fighting, eating, drinking or just making babies. Human life has to have more meaning than that. God knows it is brief!

You could begin your self-improvement campaign by analyzing muscle and its response to specific stimuli. Every muscle has the capacity to extend and contract. More than 600 muscles in your body constitute about 40% of your body weight, and they are designed to create motion of the skeletal system and directed by your nervous system. Since muscle weighs more than fat, the actuarial scales developed by insurance companies for diet recommendations and general health are totally invalid for anyone who is involved in a body-building (muscle developing) program. It is not uncommon for a male body builder to tip the scale at well over 200 lbs. with less than 10% body fat, while some trim female fitness competitors weigh close to 150. You are advised, if you use the schedule which follows, to throw away your scale and buy a few good full-length mirrors. Hang one in every room. For brutal evaluation, hang one on the ceiling above your bed. Your mate will think it is kinky!

Women body builders need not worry about developing muscle as massive as men, unless they foolishly consider injecting themselves with androgenic steroids that shut down their normal estrogen production and increase their testosterone beyond natural levels. Many professional female body builders do indeed follow that tack, because unscrupulous bodybuilding promoters have established massive muscularity as a standard of value in exchange for their coveted trophy. Their resultant masculine countenance includes other notable aberrations: Supplemental androgenic steroids, taken by women in excess, stimulate facial hair growth, deeper voices, aggressive behavior, and often create enlarged clitoris size. Of course, these developments attract some women who may have an abnormal level of the male hormone to begin with, but they are not part of the original female design. Hormonal imbalance, an accident of nature, is preponderant in the clinically homosexual community, which is why it is inconsiderate to fault them for their sexual preferences.

Our hormones must certainly be addressed as part of our defense against muscular atrophy, common among the aged, and we have included a chapter for you that offers cutting edge conjecture about hormone replacement therapy, which, we believe, will produce 21st century men and women of exceptionally powerful and energetic countenance. Even testosterone, which has taken a bad rap due to its abuse by professional bodybuilders, can be cardioproductive at optimum levels, since supplementation of testosterone dilates the arteries, as reported in *Clinical Science* (1998). There is also no doubt that testosterone therapy for aged men is indicated, due to its rapid natural decline, its drop from the Fountain of Youth, but testosterone replacement therapy alone will not get you there. Weight-resistance exercise that stresses the muscles supporting your bones will expedite the regenerating process. If truly stressed, muscles tear from weight resistance during the training period. It is during the resting period between exercise sessions that stressed muscles repair, and, as they rejuvenate, dormant muscle fibers are awakened and recruited to assist in the anticipated struggle against the next stressful resistance. This kind of empowerment will lead to muscle hypertrophy, if the weight resistance is formidable and the motion is slow. Fast-twitch muscle will respond and the muscle will enlarge, if properly fueled.

To assist in protein synthesis, energy production and hyper-development, professional bodybuilders ingest the supplement Creatine (a muscle cell volumizer), Glutamine (the most abundant amino acid in all muscle fiber), and extraordinary amounts of protein for muscle nourishment and nitrogen retention. Average bodybuilders consume at least one gram of protein for each pound of body weight; more, if they want to gain in muscular weight and size. They have proven the medical establishment of the middle of this century to be wrong in their condemnation of excess protein. A high-protein diet is compulsory for high intensity body builders to attain strength and lean mass and to avoid the dreaded waste of muscle called catabolism. Since the amount of food necessary to keep up with this process would be voluminous, distending the stomach, ionized whey protein powders are taken regularly to supplement food ingestion. The regimen encourages frequent small feedings (at least six) as opposed to the customary three meals a day, low in saturated fat, moderate in complex carbohydrates, and high in protein. Another important supplement, beta-hydroxy beta-methyl-butyrate (HMB) has been proven to guard against catabolism during the muscle repair and strengthening process. HMB is present in breast milk, a natural metabolite of the branched chain amino acid Leucine. HMB strengthens the immune system and lowers blood cholesterol. Twice the gains in strength and muscle mass can be expected from ingesting three grams a day, while aerobic capacity will also be enhanced, even among the aged. Vukovich, et. al., (1997). I take a gram with each meal. It is necessary that you understand these fueling prerequisites before embarking on your weight-training journey.

Since testosterone, the male hormone, was designed for strength and aggression, pro bodybuilders for years have injected variations of it as a supplement, along with other androgenic steroids. This practice, together with injections of a variety of diuretics taken to deplete water and promote vascularity, has raised the budget of pro bodybuilders to enormous expenditures, combined with the cost of supplemental human growth hormone and insulin. Food supplement companies usually foot the bill in exchange for testimonials that promote their product. The public is led to believe that the gargantuan proportions developed by these steroid enhanced giants resulted only from exercise and from ingestion of their protein powders. Unfortunately, the overabundant abuse of this drug regimen has caused the death of a few top-rated pros and has led to liver and kidney problems in others. Especially embarrassing to well-known "champions" of the bodybuilding community is the pencil-necked countenance to which they've returned since they stopped shooting "roids." Their reduction of lean tissue mass is compounded, if they stop high intensity workouts, often deprecated by doomsayer mainstream physicians, creating shadows of their former selves. The AMA and antiquated actuarial scales from insurance companies have convinced these former giants of their industry that thin men live longer. The resultant humiliation that follows their dramatic size reduction may be a deserved punishment for having cheated by using drugs to attain their former champion status.

With the emergence of natural substances like 19-Norandrostenediol, professional bodybuilders may win contests of the next century without injecting steroids. Steroids have become illegal in the U.S., but their debilitating side effects should be of more concern to young bodybuilders than their illegality. We implore you to have your blood checked periodically by a complementary physician before and during any diet, prohormonal or hormonal supplementation program. Surely do not consider HGH or testosterone injections, unless your levels of IGF- I and testosterone are low; if they are, see a complementary physician and go for it!

The search for natural substances to replace damaging steroids has resulted in the production of DHEA, pregnenolone, androstenedione, norandrostenediol, and the herb Tribulus Terrestris (from the plant called Crown of Thorns), all natural testosterone precursors. Mark McGwire, St. Louis Cardinals slugger who led the League in home run clouts in 1998, admitted to the use of some of testosterone precursor supplements, claiming, "Everybody I know in the game of baseball uses the same stuff I use." The latest of these over-the-counter supplements, a powerful testosterone precursor, is 19-Norandrostenediol, said to find a direct pathway to nortestosterone (Nandrolone), effectively avoiding production of dehydrotestosterone and estrogen. The former can lead to prostate enlargement, and too much estrogen in males can lead to the development of female characteristics like gynecomastia (the development of breast tissue in males). The only estrogen antagonist proven to block the conversion of testosterone to estrogen by the class of enzymes called aromatase is a substance called chrysin. If you should decide to take any testosterone booster, men, we strongly advise you to include a generous amount of Saw Palmetto or other prostate growth inhibitors, like Pygeum, in the stack, to avert prostate enlargement, and a testosterone booster that includes chrysin. Blood tests can, of course, monitor your PSA, a measure of prostate size. We must repeat that no hormone supplementation should be undertaken without a doctor's evaluation and prescription.

Exercise that does not produce hypertrophy or enlargement of muscle, but does tax and improve your oxygen supply, enhancing your endurance, as we have mentioned, is called aerobic. It must be constant, but not stressful, for a minimum of 30 minutes (for fat reduction and arterial diameter dilation), and should be interrupted with at least one-high intensity sprint for a minimum of 30 seconds. Inclusion of 3 or 4 of these sprints during the 30 minutes of steady low-intensity activity is the most effective waist slimmer, especially if the exercise is before breakfast. These exercises develop slow-twitch muscle fibers, many of which are also anxiously dormant in the human who is lethargic. These fibers can be developed and maintained through obviously aerobic activities like walking, jogging, and the latest vogue, spinning, but also can be trained with weight resistance, if the rest periods between exercises are minimal. Any constant slow body motion for a minimum of 30 minutes, interrupted with 30 seconds of intense activity, may be considered beneficial aerobic exercise, categorized as high intensity interval training (HIIT). Professional bodybuilders must include aerobic exercises in their weekly regimen to burn subcutaneous fat and reveal muscular definition. Some dismiss aerobic exercise as an unnecessary expenditure of time, gaining just as much benefit from adding a final set of 100 low-weight repetitions to each exercise of their daily program, another very efficient technique. I prefer to alternate this approach with HIIT, which whittled my waist in just 12 weeks (see Figs. 64a and 64b), enhanced by avoidance of beer, sugar, starch and carbonated sodas, and flushed with plenty of water.

The 30-minute imperative was born from research which reveals the exercise energy source for the first 15 constant minutes as glycogen (sugar). We begin to burn fat at the 16th minute of constant activity. Exercisers who jump onto a treadmill for 15 minutes or less are wasting their time, if fat reduction is their goal. We see many at our Sugarbush Sports Complex who carry the same fat they had when they began two or three years ago. Bodybuilders who train with weights are fat-burning engines, which continue to idle when they are at rest, since their muscles are repairing at that time. The process is thermogenic, and heat burns calories. All day.

Since total development of physical potential is our goal, we have recently elected to combine some aerobic activity with at least a few days of anaerobic training, working different body parts each exercise day, i.e., Monday: biceps, triceps, and forearms; Wednesday: thighs and calves; Friday: upper back and shoulders; Sunday: chest and lower back, Tuesday: repeat schedule of previous Monday, including a rest day between each gym visit. Such a workout schedule requires no more than an hour in the gym, with plenty of rest time for the repair of each muscle area. We begin at least two of those workouts with 30 minutes of treadmill walking, interrupted by three or four 30-second sprints. Younger readers might consider fewer rest days, but are advised to not follow an arm day with an exercise that includes arm movement. Thus, thighs and calves on Tuesday could follow arms on Monday, followed by upper back and shoulders Wednesday, and a rest day Thursday. Friday could be a chest day, and so on.

Our female readers need not worry about developing masculine looking bodies from following such a routine, unless your hormones are out of balance. You will just become more shapely, more attractive, and certainly more functional, since the exigencies of life at the close of this century demand a strong countenance. If you doubt this claim, you are probably not living. Living your life and not merely existing for the comfort of others means taking part in the adventures that life offers. Some people receive pleasure from watching the Discovery Channel, while others discover. Some buy calendars illustrated with beautiful mountain scenes, while others climb and ski those majestic slopes. You may think you have been living, but living implies performing. With a body that is fit, you will look forward to adventure.

Less adventurous demands for strength including the lifting of babies, the moving of furniture, the acrobatics of making love (if your mate is not a necrophiliac), to say nothing of life's emergencies that call for your physical response. When you dismiss strength as an unnecessary requirement of humanity, you dismiss the living of life; you are cheating yourself and programming your senior years as the part of your life doomed to suffer through devastating debilitation, a burden for those whom you have raised and to whom you have given so much. The choice is yours. Of course, if you are morbidly obese or fast approaching that status, you probably find the short walk to your car a challenging feat of strength. Get rid of some of that fat before you consider high intensity exercise or you might trigger a heart attack.

The Origin of Body Fat and the Fastest Way to Lose It

Brainwashed by the delusion that fat ingestion is the primary cause of obesity, our nation is currently on a zero-fat craze. Low fat or zero fat are the principal claims on the labels of just about every supermarket item. Yet, citizens have lost not a pound and many of you are obviously getting fatter. W.C. Willett, in the 1998 *American Journal of Clinical Nutrition*, claims that truth is that low fat consumption, up to 40% of the total daily diet, has very little effect upon total body mass. It is time to challenge the fat-phobic nutritional fallacy and reconsider the proclamation offered by Dr. Robert Atkins over two decades ago.

Although fat may contain higher calories, it also produces satiety soon after ingestion. The real problem with the American diet is our addiction to sugar, simple carbohydrates. Excessive ingestion of sweets trigger a flood of insulin from the pancreas. Surplus insulin goes beyond response to the ingested sugar into the bloodstream, devouring your normal blood sugar levels and causing the chronic fatigue syndrome called hypoglycemia. Since satiety does not follow sugar ingestion, the sugar addict will crave more sugar to fight a low blood sugar fatigued condition.

Excess ingestion of simple carbohydrate is stored in adipose tissue and in your circulatory system as debilitating triglycerides; it is a natural defense system to store energy for the primitive days, when food was not bountiful. Any sugar ingested that goes beyond the quantity that your brain needs for fuel is stored as fat. This is really what you are wearing and there is only one fast way to lose it: Deprive yourself of all carbohydrates for a short period of time, eating all the protein you can consume (up to 45 grams at one sitting) and drinking lots of water. You will soon go into a state of ketosis, wherein your brain, in being deprived of carbohydrates for its fuel, will go to your own fat deposits for its need. At that moment, you will become a fat-burning engine instead of a sugar-driven machine, and fat (your own fat) is a much more efficient fuel.

Many readers go no farther when they peruse Dr. Atkins' theory and condemn this diet of zero carbohydrate and ketosis as dangerous. Let us clear the air. At no time has the brilliant cardiologist recommended zero carbohydrates as a permanent nutritional regimen. What he has suggested is that each of us has a particular limit for carbohydrate ingestion, and that when that level is exceeded, the excess sugar will be stored as fat. This is not the conjecture of some self-accredited nutritionist; this is medical fact, offered by a qualified heart specialist. It would be a good idea for you to know what your specific tolerance level is. You can, with a very simple self-administered test.

Dr. Atkins advises you to pick up a jar of Ketostix at any drug store for testing your urine. Begin the temporary zero carbohydrate diet, testing your urine with one of the Ketostix daily. Eat all the protein you wish, but keep each ingestion under 45 grams for optimum digestion. Frequent small portions are preferred to gluttonous huge meals; this includes seafood, chicken, veal, pork, and lean beef, plus eggs, and a good modicum of hard cheeses (like Locatelli Romano, our favorite). You truly need not worry about eating the yolks, as the Lord has placed a sufficient amount of lecithin in egg yolk to emulsify its cholesterol. While no one has ever proven that the ingestion of cholesterol can cause your blood serum cholesterol to rise significantly, only patients with a history of cholesterolemia need limit their ingestion of the yolk of an egg, one of nature's most perfect foods. Drink at least ten glasses of water a day. You may even eat one bowl of lettuce each day, as its carbohydrate content is negligible. Pour some olive oil over it liberally (it is a healthy unsaturated fat). Frank takes a high-potency multiple vitamin and mineral tablet each day, along with multiple antioxidants that include at least 400 iu of vitamin E, 50 mcg of selenium, 3 grams of vitamin C, and 30 mg of Pycnogenol. Phosphatidyl choline, 420 mg, is a high-potency lecithin that has given Frank vital energy while on this diet. He also claims that 360 mg of EPA and 240 mg of DHA, fish oil supplements, have revved his new engine, as has 1000 mg of flaxseed. Another oil energy stimulant, called medium chain triglycerides (MCT), available in most health food stores, is very popular among professional bodybuilders. These oils are essential for the effectiveness of Dr. Atkins' preferred ketogenic diet, as they provide fuel for energy to accompany the energy you will get from burning your own stored fat.

After several days of carbohydrate restriction, the Ketostix strip will begin to turn purple. When it is totally purple, which can take two weeks for some people, less time for others, the Ketostix strip is announcing that you are now in a state of ketosis. Your brain has begun to fuel itself from your own fat deposits; you begin to devour your own fat. You can expect to lose at least ten pounds in a few weeks; but this is just the beginning.

Next, put back some "good" carbohydrates into your diet, increasing the quantity 5 grams a week. By "good" carbs, we mean complex carbohydrates, like green vegetables, nuts and some fruit. You will need a booklet listing carbohydrate levels of various foods and will be surprised to find, for example, that a whole bowl of spinach has only 2 grams of carbohydrate, as does a delicious plum. You'll learn that a banana has 15 grams of carbohydrate, that melon is low, but pears and grapes are high. The first week of carbohydrate adding, ingest only 5 grams of carbohydrate daily; next week bump it to 10 grams; the following week 15 grams, and so on.

Keep checking your urine. The Ketostix strip will become less purple, as you approach your maximum tolerance level. When you check the strip and it is no longer purple, it is announcing that you have exceeded your limit. Simply back up 5 grams to know exactly what your carbohydrate tolerance level is. If you want to be lean, do not exceed that level for the rest of your life. Some of you will have a generous carb tolerance, perhaps 150 grams. Some, like Frank, will have an exceptionally low tolerance level of 60 grams daily. If you ingest 5 grams more than your tolerance level, you can rest assured that those 5 grams will be stored as body fat. Sugar is its origin. Sugar is your poison. Starch is converted to sugar that can even be worse for you, if you have a wheat intolerance Your stomach will distend. Drop some white bread into a glass of water and watch it swell, if you want a clue to one cause of that flesh that spills over your belt.

Here is another bonus: Go to that occasional party or social function and pig out on pizza, pie, and ice cream, until it sickens you. Then, follow that day with three days of zero carbohydrates and you will be able to tolerate the insult you inflicted upon yourself. Do not do this too often, though, as pig-out parties are for pigs.

Remember, our book does not prescribe. What we have described is the Dr. Atkins carbohydrate restriction diet that one of the authors, Frank, has found to be most effective for him. It is the diet that wise professional body builders adopt three weeks before entering a contest, to lower their body fat. It is the diet most prescribed for hypoglycemic patients and diabetics and has a history of lowering cholesterol counts and high blood pressure. It is a diet that does not restrict food quantity and in fact recommends frequent daily feedings. In fact, it is a diet that never fails. Most importantly, it is the only diet recommended by a qualified cardiologist (most nutritionists have no medical degree), and finally, it is the diet recommended by the authors of this book to fuel the exercise program that will soon follow.

You would do well to eliminate refined sugar entirely. Your prehistoric cousins did not need it. Refined sugar in this country is less than 200 years old, curiously parallel to the rise in atherosclerotic mortality. Sugar is referred to as a simple carbohydrate, and its debilitating influence is the same, whether you get it from hard candy or from excessive fruit and its juices. Consider the blubber that characterizes many Hawaiians, whose staple food is fruit, "simple" carbohydrate; the "energy" it produces may be quick, but is not lasting. The body fat sugar produces is obvious. Take another look at your sugarholic friends. Sugar triggers your pancreas to churn out insulin explosively, but that insulin attacks the sugar in your blood, lowering it significantly; your momentary, high or jolt of energy comes crashing down, screaming "more...more.. more." And that cry is usually accommodated. The state of chronic fatigue that eventually follows, called hypoglycemia, is the most common affliction of our society as we close this century, with diabetes waiting anxiously in the wings.

The sugar industry would have you believe that fat is the primary killer. History does not support this conjecture. Fat and protein were the primary foods of primitive man and are still staples in the vast Tundra, where no cases of atherosclerosis have been found among the Eskimo community. At least, not until their young people move to a cosmopolitan city like Anchorage and discover sugar and processed foods. Of course, we all love sugar; we were raised with sugar as a reward for good behavior. Our parents had no idea that reward would become a debilitating addiction. Many grandparents still buy love from their precious grandchildren with lollipops and candy, creating grand kids as sugar addicts before they reach puberty. Like other addictions, frequent sugar consumption soon becomes habitual. Kick the habit. It is pure poison. Remember, you are truly what you eat.

Saturated fat ingestion might be okay for industry-free Arctic Circle Eskimos, but there is no doubt that it is a pollution magnet for cosmopolitan inhabitants, one that can cause serious damage to your circulatory system from attacking free radicals if not protected with a generous daily consumption of antioxidants like vitamin C, E and the proanthocyanidins like grapeseed oil and Pycnogenol. Since prolonged heavy exercise that tears muscle also can cause damaging oxidation, potent amounts of these supplements must be considered by anyone involved in a weight-resistance program. While you might be smart enough to avoid saturated fat, you may still inadvertently ingest some with your protein, if that protein comes from red meat or some seafood.

There are good fats, though. Unsaturated fats can produce energy that is more efficient than sugar energy, since it lasts a good deal longer, i.e., fatty acids like linolenic and linoleic, fish oil fats, and the protective oil called E. Primitive man was a fat-burning engine. During the Ice Age, he was a carnivore, as evidenced by our "canine" teeth, but prehistoric animals were not always easy to catch, so he fished. Even when the ice melted, when game was lean and the fish were not biting, he ate leaves, from which hc ingested herbs, fruit and nuts. Ginko Biloba may have nourished his brain, Saw Palmetto probably kept his prostate from growing, while leaves from the bush we call the "Crown of Thorns" (Tribulus Terrestris) and wild yams, from which comes DHEA, stoked his testosterone. Herbs like Guarana and Ma Huang gave him explosive energy, and willow bark (from which we get aspirin) kept his blood thin. We are only 10,000 years from that period of time. Farming is only 8000 years old. Food processing has barely passed one century.

With farming, of course, came a preponderance of complex carbohydrates like corn, carrots, wheat and barley, potatoes and rice. Woman learned to grind meal; it kept her mate home longer. Man, overwhelmed by the size and strength of his animal food sources, began to hunt less, farm more, eat more carbohydrates and propagate more, with more leisure and less time required for the "hunt." With these diet changes came a dramatic change in blood type. DNA testing of prehistoric man remains prior to the farming period suggests that the original blood type was O. Perhaps this is the reason that Type O recipients can donate blood to anyone, whereas other blood types can only give to others of their blood type and could also mean that we, who have Type O blood, have low tolerance for carbohydrates.

Important to consider is that carbohydrates were originally ingested by man as a supplement to his primarily protein and fat diet, certainly not as his primary food source. This is strong evidence against the ape-to-man evolution theory. We are a different species. Of interest, also, is to compare the tall skeletons of the Ice Age man with prehistoric remains of shorter cadavers from the later farming period. The Ice Age era, the protein and fat diet period, produced men and women of thick bone and, as we have noted elsewhere, stronger muscle (indicated by the areas of bone where muscle was connected). Ice Agers were muscular, and apparently, stood taller than the farming humanoids who were to follow. Ice Age people had better teeth and powerful muscles; compare them to the chubby Hawaiians of today who live on fruit, juices and simple carbohydrates. Face it, your body fat came from sugar. You refuse to acknowledge this evidence because you love the taste. Sugarholics live in the same denial abyss as their unfortunate alcoholic neighbors. They would rather die than give up pie.

So, to fuel your body and health improvement schedule, you might want to look seriously at Frank's adopted high-protein, moderate complex carbohydrates, low saturated fat (if you are not living at the North Pole), zero simple carbohydrate and adequate essential fatty acid diet. (Remember, we are not prescribing, but merely reporting the regimen of one individual.)

In addition, Frank gave up all carbonated soft drinks that bloat your stomach. Also dismissed by him is milk, except for children, and processed cheese, while his water volume has dramatically increased. Adequate daily consumption for healthy blood and organs should be around 100 ounces of water daily for a 200-lb. man; that translates to a minimum of 12 eight- ounce glasses per day. Ease into this regimen, though, or you will be urinating all night. Most people do not drink enough water, one of God's most precious gifts. Frank has watched his son, Mark, living away from him for 16 years, and therefore not under his guidance, go through an entire day without water. Like so many teens he was addicted to sodas. A recent custody exchange has dramatically improved Mark's health, as Barbara Covino keeps no beverage but water in her refrigerator. Sound familiar? The current American public drenches thirst with sodas, beer and booze, every liquid but the one God intended for us to drink. If you wonder why Man develops illnesses that his animal cousins do not, you only have to watch what both species eat and drink. Man blames his illnesses upon "old age." Age does not create atherosclerosis, cancer, osteoporosis; foolish habits do. Man has shortened his own life expectancy by changing the fuel that the Lord provided for active longevity, and, do you recall from Genesis, the "forbidden fruit" was sugar. All fruit is sugar under colorful skins, and we are all descendants of Eve.

A moderate amount of complex carbs will provide the natural glycogen energy that muscles need to combat weight resistance. We get our carbs from whole grain breads (as little as possible), green leaf vegetables (the yellow vegetables high in carbohydrate content), potato skins (we discard the starch-laden rest), wild rice, and oat bran (5000 mg a day will lower anyone's cholesterol). All other carbohydrates in our diet come from food supplements like protein powder and high-performance Creatine; the latter includes carbohydrates to trigger an insulin discharge, which rushes the Creatine to the muscle cells. Dr. Paul Greenhaff of the School of Biomedical Sciences at Queens Medical Center in Nottingham, England reports a 6.6% higher concentration of Creatine in the muscle of test subjects who included a carbohydrate with their creatine supplement, when compared to those who took Creatine alone; 75 grams of carbohydrate with 5 or 6 grams of Creatine seems to work best.

It has been recommended in their trade magazines that bodybuilders should ingest one gram of protein for every pound of body weight to increase strength, more for massive muscular development. The current Mr. Olympia ingests 300 grams of protein daily. To get that much protein from food would necessitate huge volumes of meat, fish, and poultry, grossly distending the stomach. (We can see this quite clearly in the super heavyweight bodies of Olympic weight lifters, in the portly bodies of the World's Strongest Man contestants, and in some gluttonous professional wrestlers.) If their beer-barrel silhouette amuses you and is far from the symmetrical ideal you envision as your goal, you must supplement your diet with ionized whey protein powders, easily accessible today from any health food store and in better supermarkets and drug stores (ionized whey derivation is best). Since small frequent meals are better for constant energy and to avoid stomach distention, one strategy the bodybuilding champions follow is to include a high-protein drink at some hour between breakfast and lunch, another between lunch and dinner, and still another at bedtime. If their goal is to gain weight, they would choose a drink supplement that includes a high level of carbohydrate along with a minimum of 34 grams of protein. Do not overdo the protein in one course. The maximum amount of protein that can be digested at one time is 45 grams. To lose weight, we would choose a drink with a similar protein level but close to zero carbohydrates. All drink supplements should include close to zero fat content.

For energy, dieting chubbies who adopt a high-protein, low-carbohydrate regimen, can get plenty from medium chain triglycerides (MCT) oils available at most health food stores, and from Octocosanol, a vitamin E product highly recommended by Dr. Robert Atkins. Other excellent fats for energy can come from olive oil, flaxseed, safflower oil, and in the gamma linoleic oil of the evening primrose. We also prefer whey protein drinks that include the most abundant amino acid in muscle, <u>glutamine</u>. Bodybuilders are advised to ingest 10 to 15 grams of glutamine daily to avoid catabolism (muscle tissue deterioration); 3 or 4 grams of Phosphatidyl Serine is another important cortisol-protective supplement after a bout of exercise that was intense enough to tear muscle tissue. Finally, some high-protein drinks include HMB and an abundance of branched chain amino acids (BCAA's) for muscle resynthesis after stress.

Bodybuilders who are striving for maximum muscle size with low body fat have learned that such size (admittedly assisted by androgenic steroids) must be led with high protein <u>and</u> high carbohydrates (of the complex variety, not simple sugars). Some bodybuilders load great volumes of complex carbohydrates on weekends and switch to zero carbs during the week. Others pig out on carbs for two weeks and then follow with two weeks of zero carbs. Both systems are <u>highly anaerobic</u> for massive development of lean tissue devoid of fat. You do not need foods made from refined sugar; these are simple carbohydrates that will hasten your aging and cause a variety of debilitating diseases. Kick the habit. It is not too late. So much for the fuel. Now let us learn how to expend it.

Exercises for the Physically Challenged

You know who you are. You have not moved with any amount of real stress since you were forced to in Military Basic Training, or by your Phys. Ed. teacher in high school. Your car, your taxi, or your subway has become one of your extremities, an extension of your foot. You have worked hard at maintaining a home and raising children and feel you get "enough exercise." Or, you have been so loyal to your corporation, you have had no time for exercise and you are certainly too exhausted to exercise after work, so the couch has become still another extremity, an attachment, replete with TV remote control. You are plagued with chronic fatigue and vulnerable to every virus that waits patiently on every subway strap and every doorknob. You are probably fat or anorexic from lack of optimum nutrition and excess consumption of smoke. You are secretly pleased that your mate is also falling apart, as it gives you license to reject the notion that self-improvement is within your reach; why "get in shape" when your mate is pitifully out of it? The few mirrors in your home are small, reflecting only your face. You do not fear old age, but welcome it, as you can then revert to adolescence and have others care for you. You dote on your children, lest they not feel obligated to care for you in your senior years. This age of political correctness would label you "the physically challenged" Mr. and Mrs. Average American.

While we refuse to prescribe for anyone we have not personally evaluated, we provide for you here an outline of exercises similar to those devised by Frank years ago for his chapter, "Prepare Yourself," an introduction to his 1976 book, *Skiers Digest.* Since these body-strengthening movements require no weights, they therefore may be regarded as less demanding of extreme stress for the physically challenged. Each of the major muscles will be isolated, defined, and matched to a particular exercise for development of strength and hypertrophy. Three months after beginning the schedule outlined by Frank, any participant will be ready for the next phase: Muscular development from progressive weight resistance, which will follow this initiation.

While these first exercises require no iron resistance, you may be required to solicit the assistance of a friend or your mate. Perhaps you are lucky enough to have both in the same person. You will both benefit. Muscular development of any part of your body is dependent upon the stress involved from your resistance to an opposing force and upon the amount of time that muscle is subjected to the necessary tension. The program will involve sets of a number of repetitions. Every workout session should begin with a warm-up to prevent cramping. Let us begin with the muscles that support your head, the sternocleidomastoids. Attached to your sternum and to the bones behind your ears, these are the whiplash protectors. If you can't see yours, get your thyroid checked; you may have a goiter. Frank calls the exercise a migraine mender.

DAY ONE

Start every exercise with a "warm-up." Best is a 25-repetition set of the exercise that will follow with little resistance.

The Migraine Mender. The sternocleidomastoid muscles flank the larynx, connected to the sternum (the dagger-like bone

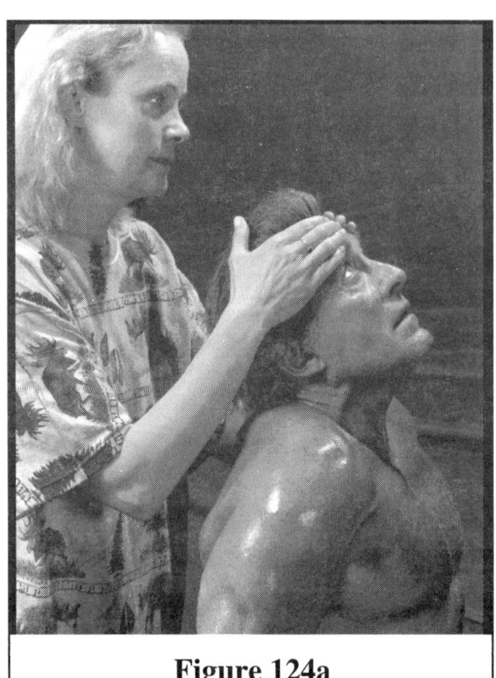

Figure 124a

Barbi provides resistance for Frank's Migraine Mender exercise.

that separates your ribs in the center of your chest), and to the bones behind your ears called the mastoid. Exercise of this important head-supporting muscle will flush your brain with nourishing blood, alleviating headaches and protecting you from whiplash events.

All muscles have antagonistic muscles which act in reverse, when a muscle contracts, its antagonistic partner extends, and vice versa. To avoid binding or shortening of a muscle length, it is wise to follow a set of contraction exercises with a set of extensions which contract their opposing antagonists. In counterpoint to the sternocleidomastoid muscles are the two heads of the trapezius at the rear of the base of the skull. Thus, when the sternocleidomastoids contract, the heads of the trapezius extend; when this top part of the trapezius contracts, the sternocleidomastoids extends.

For strength and development of the sternocleidomastoids the head must move forward and downward against resistance. Begin with a "warm-up" set of 25 repetitions against imagined resistance before 3 sets of 10 repetitions against real resistance. A workout partner can assist in providing this resistance by standing behind you and clasping hands on your forehead. As you work your neck muscles, your partner can work their biceps and pectorals by resisting the movement of your head forward and downward (Fig. 124a). You are advised

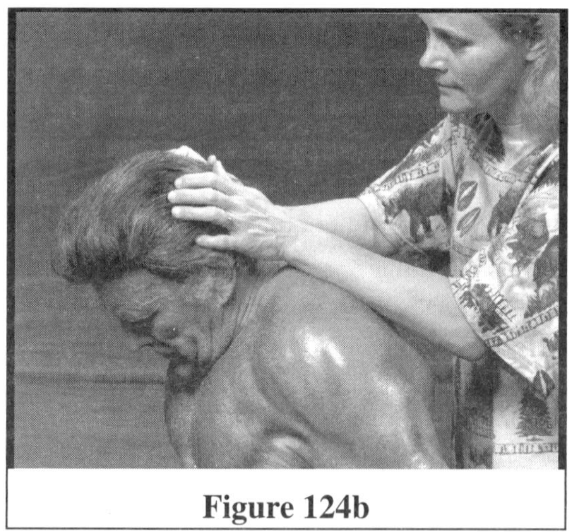

Figure 124b

Negative resistance against return movement builds strength and protects against whiplash.

to stretch your head upward before each forward movement. For maximum amount of time under muscle stressing tension, take ten seconds to contract, exerting maximum force against the resistance. Hold the contraction for a count of one. Then take five seconds to return. For "negative" resistance on the return, your partner can switch hands to the back of your head and press lightly against your rear movement (Fig. 124b). This negative return is called "eccentric"; it will warm up your trapezius for the second exercise.

Whiplash. A common injury to passengers when an automobile "stops short" is compression of vertebral discs in the cervical area. A C6 fracture could sever the spinal cord and cause paralysis. Well-developed upper heads of the trapezius muscle could protect against this. For resistance, you can use an ordinary towel and your own arm strength. Bend forward as you sit on a chair. Place the towel behind your head, grasping its end with each hand. Pull downward until your chin touches your clavicle. To exercise the upper heads of the trapezius, apply head pressure against the towel as you roll your head upward and back, resisting the action by pulling the towel downward with your hands (Fig. 125a). To warm-up, apply little pull, to permit 15 to 25 repetitions. Then, perform 3 sets of 10 repetitions, following the same slow cadence as before: 10 seconds of contraction, applying maximum counter resistance with the towel; a one-second hold against full resistance; and a five-second

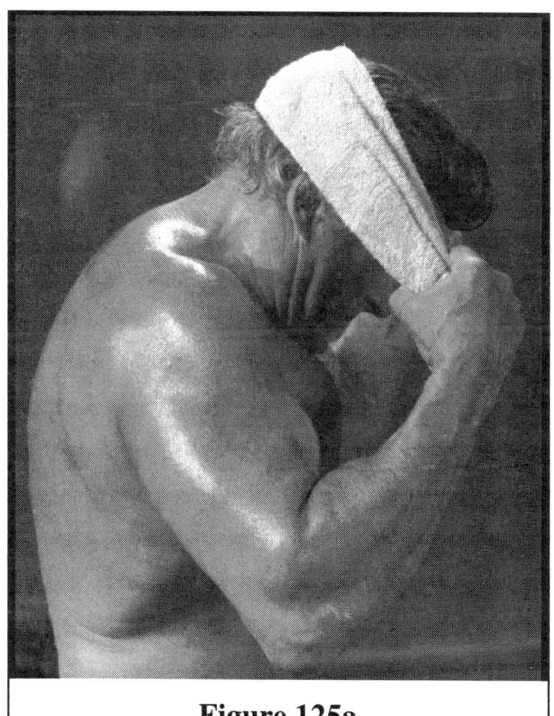

Figure 125a

A towel replaces Barbi for those workouts without a partner.

slow return, for each repetition. Your face will flush from the rush of blood to these muscles that support the skull. A surge of mental energy usually follows these first two exercises and headaches magically disappear.

The blood you have summoned to volumize the cells within the stressed muscles will create a swelling and tightness throughout your neck. Bodybuilders call this a "burn," a gratifying announcement that you have performed the exercise properly, and with sufficient rest, strength and muscular development of the stressed area will ensue. Do not minimize the importance of rest. As explained earlier, no muscle develops during exercise. Muscle is, in fact, torn during that stress. If sufficient rest follows (three days for younger, stronger readers, four days to a week for us old timers) dormant muscle fibers are recruited as the stressed muscle repairs, to assist resistance against future stress; this is a natural survival mechanism. The process is accelerated if 45 grams of protein and at least 75 grams of carbohydrate are ingested, along with 5 grams of Creatine, within a 2-hour window right after an exercise session.

The supplement Creatine has been proven to be a safe energy and strength supplier, a cell volumizer with no side effects, if ingestion is not excessive. Supplementing with Creatine is like eating a few steaks, without the fat and cattle injected steroids, and, of course, without mass food volume to stretch your stomach. No professional athlete would dare to compete without the assistance of this important supplement in these last years of the 20th century. Most companies that produce Creatine (the best substance comes from Germany) advise a loading phase of 20 grams a day for 5 to 7 days, followed by a daily dose of 5 grams, cycling one week off every month. Stagger the ingestion during the loading phase. Creatine supplementation will increase body weight and muscular size due to muscle cell volumization. Do not watch the scale; instead, get friendly with the mirror.

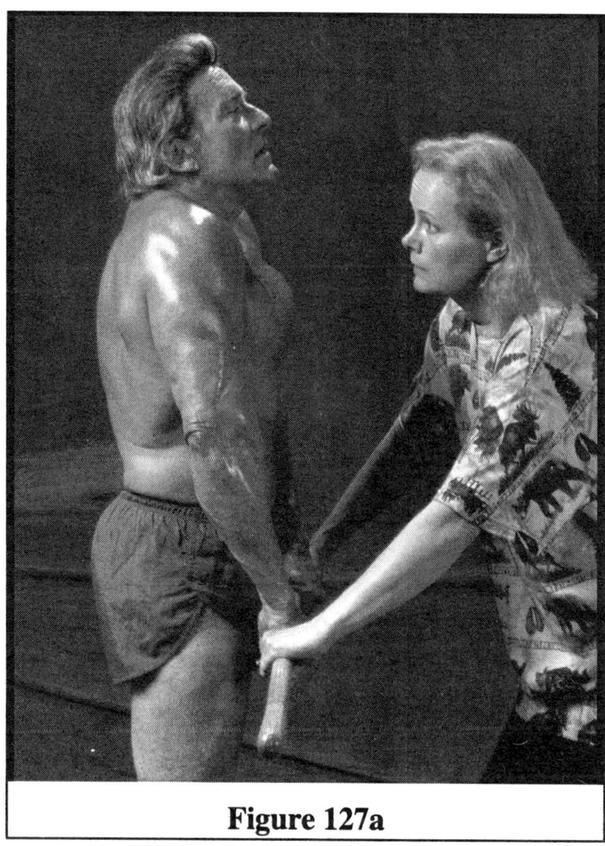

Figure 127a

A workout partner can apply sufficient resistance to a hand-held bar for trap shrugs.

Trap Tugging. With your blood having been urgently summoned to your neck, exercise of a neighboring muscular area is advisable next, as it will already have been partially warmed. Shaped like a kite (hence its label trapezius) the principal muscle of the upper back assists in the lifting of heavy objects from the ground. Its contraction is effected by "shrugging," lifting the shoulders toward the ears. For resistance, use a 3- or 4- foot dowel or pipe, which your partner can press down as you attempt to shrug (Fig. 127a). Your grip should, of course, be centered, about a shoulder width apart; your partner's grip should be wider, to allow for full movement. With your arms fully extended, tilt your chin up, chest inflated, and tug by lifting the resistance with only your trapezius muscle, raising your shoulders to your ears. Do 3 sets of ten repetitions, with a cadence of 10-1-5 (10 seconds to contract, one second to hold and squeeze at apogee, and 5 seconds to descend). Allow no more than a 3 minute rest between sets.

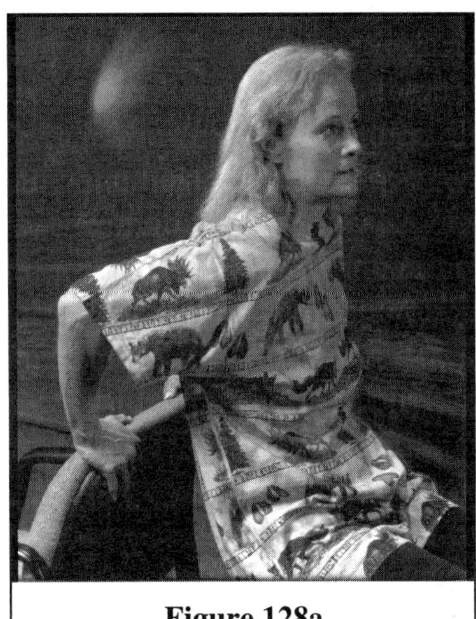

Figure 128a

Until you get stronger, table-edge dips will develop triceps and pectoral strength.

Cheater Dips. As an antagonist to trap tugs, dips offer the added benefit of triceps and pectoral development; advanced bodybuilders perform these between parallel bars, with an extra weight suspended from a belt around their waist. For the physically challenged, the edge of a table may be used (Fig. 128a). Move your feet forward to allow your hips to drop until your arms contract to a right angle; this motion contracts the trapezius and extends the triceps of your arms, stretching also the pectoral muscles of your chest. Slowly press against the table edge, taking 10 seconds to extend. Do not lock your elbows at the point of apogee, but, just before that point, tense your triceps and hold their contraction for a count of one second (Fig. 128b). Then, take 5 seconds to descend. Try for 3 sets of 10 reps; if you find this difficult, even 6 repetitions should be beneficial. If 6 are difficult, you are woefully weak and may rest assured that your triceps are close to

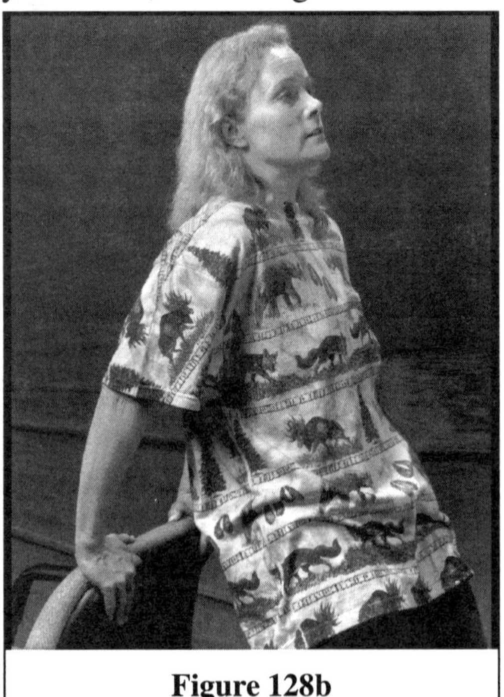

Figure 128b

Time under tension produces strength and development.

mortal atrophy. It may not be too late to change that. Try to "cheat" by not descending as low as specified. Descend only a few inches, until you are strong enough to drop 6 inches. Eventually, you will become strong enough to perform the exercise as initially described. When you are ready to go beyond cheater dips, try the exercise with your hands on one bench and your feet on another.

These four upper body exercises are all you need for your day's first encounter, if you are among the physically challenged. These exercises are anaerobic and designed for muscular strength and development. Schedule 30 minutes tomorrow for aerobic activity.

DAY TWO

If one of your goals is to lose body fat, I recommend performance of your aerobic exercise before breakfast. With less carbohydrate in your system to draw upon for energy, your own fat will become your engine, and, as it is expended, so will it be depleted, with no recently ingested sugar to take its place. Aerobic exercise is not just for the obese, however. Anaerobic training will build muscle, but the inclusion of an aerobic regimen in anyone's exercise program will dilate your arteries for efficient blood flow and will probably extend your life expectancy, as the diameter of your arteries will increase.

For a jolt of energy before a workout, I have not found any better stimulant than a stack of ephedrine (in the natural form of Ma Huang), caffeine (in the natural form of Guarana), and aspirin (in the natural form of White Willow Bark Extract). There are several commercial products available in good health foods stores which include this stack in their proper ratios. Leading brands are Thermadrene, Xenadrine, and Twin Lab's Diet Fuel. Slender individuals should only consider half the amount, if any at all, since you already have a high metabolism and are naturally thermogenic.

Ma Huang is a natural herb used by Chinese physicians for over five centuries to cure asthma, hay fever, and other bronchial conditions. It contains alkaloids like ephedrine, pseudoephedrine, and norephedrine (referred to as phenylpropanolamine). Most allergy and cold medicines contain these ingredients to clear nasal passages and to cure shortness of breath. Ma Huang has a long history of safe use, if it has not been overdosed. Americans have consumed over one billion doses of ephedra products over the past five years; their safety has been assured by such qualified physicians as Stephen Edward

Kimme, M.D., M.S., F.A.C.C., assistant Professor of Cardiovascular Medicine at the University of Pennsylvania, and Steven B. Larch, M.D., nationally renowned toxicologist and athlete death investigator.

According to D.G. Bell, et al. (1998), the combination of Ma Huang with caffeine-based products has been proven to extend and stimulate athletic performance, probably due to hyper stimulation of the central nervous system and to the conversion of sugar burning engines to fat burning machines.

Be cautious of commercial weight-reducing products; some, which combine ephedrine and caffeine with yohimbine, are heart bursters. These products increase blood pressure and raise the heart rate, while decreasing the blood-pumping efficiency of the heart. Since an ephedrine/caffeine stack has no such effect upon the heart when used alone or with aspirin, yohimbine is deduced to be the adverse ingredient (Waluga, M., et al., "Cardiovascular effects of ephedrine, caffeine and yohimbine measures by thoracic, electrical and bioimpedance in obese women", *Clinical Physiology*, 1998).

Caffeine, preferably in the form of Guarana, helps to liberate fatty acids from adipose tissue, increasing our ability to "burn fat"; it certainly increases focus, endurance, and possibly strength during any workout. Synergistically enhanced with a minimum of 10% Ma Huang, there is no more effective natural thermogenic stimulant. Natural prostaglandins, however, will try to counteract this resultant rise of body temperature. Hence, our proposed inclusion of aspirin (ASA) in its natural herbal form, White Willow Bark Extract, will complete the energy-producing stack, effectively blocking the protective prostaglandins.

Our reason for proposing herbal stacks rather than the specific drugs ephedrine, caffeine, and aspirin, is to avoid the unpleasant side effects that frequently follow the use of these drugs: high blood pressure, tremors, insomnia, and speed-like anxiety. Commercial aspirin can also cause some gastronomical damage in some individuals, which can be avoided by using its herbal equivalent, White Willow Bark Extract.

As we have defined it, aerobic activity is any oxygen-demanding action of the body that continues for a minimum of 30 minutes at 75% of your maximum heart rate, with no interruption other than an optional increased effort during spurts, or sprints, sufficient to raise the heart beat to above 75% of the maximum heart rate. Your primary energy for aerobic exercise comes from the oxidation or burning of fats and carbohydrates. Increased respiration draws in more oxygen as the heart rate increases; this also invites damaging free radicals, which must be resisted by ingestion of antioxidants like vitamin E and Pycnogenol.

The heart rate also increases along with respiration during anaerobic activity to an even higher degree, but the primary energy source for anaerobic exercise, like weight-resistance movement, is adenosine triphosphate (ATP) and creatine phosphate, especially if the muscles are stressed against formidable resistance like weights. Concomitant with this type of energy source is the accumulation of waste materials like ammonia, carbon and lactic acid in the muscles and in the blood, all of which are burned by the intake of new oxygen during the recovery period.

Examples of aerobic exercise include walking, long-distance running, cycling and competitive swimming; anaerobic activities are weight lifting, sprinting, and recreational skiing. Every turn of a recreational skier on packed terrain begins with a one-legged, downhill knee bend and pylometric spring into the "fall line." Cross-training, combining aerobic sports with anaerobic weight-resistance training, is highly recommended for life-fulfilling active longevity. As we reach the age of 40, the reductive difference in the power, stamina, and flexibility of most Americans becomes painfully obvious. Lethargy lures. Since the age of 13, Dr. Anderson has been actively involved in weight training, initially wanting to bulk up and then, as the years went by, to maintain his size along with good muscle tone and the feeling of well-being. In his 40s, he recognized a natural decrease in his power, stamina and flexibility and moreover, began to notice the loss of mental energy and the lack of discipline in wanting to work out; it was no longer fun. At this point, Dr. Anderson decided to look into the martial arts. Various DoJo's were interviewed by the doctor. He spoke with the Masters to decide with whom he wanted to study. For cross-training, he chose martial arts and weightlifting. Masters of Martial Arts, just like other professions, have certain personalities and qualities that attract or repel their students. Dr. Anderson was looking for someone balanced in both skill and spirit, someone who could motivate him along his new journey to the pinnacle of physical fitness.

Along the way while weightlifting, Dr. Anderson had been involved in sports like football, baseball, swimming, tennis, skiing, bicycling and horseback riding. Each of these sports had been adventures that he enjoyed at various stages in his life, but now, except for horseback riding and downhill skiing (neither of which could keep him in year-round ultimate shape), he was ready to move on.

After numerous interviews at various DoJo's, Dr. Anderson came upon Master David Quinlan. Talking with him and observing his various lessons delivered to students of all ages, he knew Quinlan would be the one to take him on his martial arts journey. Observing him perform the various forms of kempo/kung fu was inspiring, as the Master had an internal energy, a "life force" that Dr. Anderson needed to ignite within himself. With weightlifting, he felt he had reached a plateau of development. Visits to the gym became perfunctory. He was not motivated, neither mentally nor physically. In martial arts, the limit is endless and your goals become infinite. The many benefits obtained from martial arts include increased range of motion and flexibility, cardiovascular conditioning, increase of muscle tone, and a sense of well-being. Also, depending on the form of martial arts one chooses, you become quite skilled in self-defense, which enhances your confidence in this crazy world that we live in. Maintaining our mental capabilities also becomes a challenge as we age, and, by studying the martial arts, with its meditation, discipline, and the need to commit to memory the various forms and defense techniques, one is constantly "tweaking" the brain for renewed stimulation and recall.

One goal from cross-training is protection from the wear and tear of repetitive motions on our joints as we age. Weightlifting thickens our muscle fibers and protects the density of our bones, while martial arts gives us additional mental enhancement through meditation and cardiopulmonary stamina through rhythm controlled breathing. Weightlifting can create a strong and beautiful body. Martial arts teaches defense of that body against adversarial attack.

To obtain the most benefit from martial arts training, Dr. Anderson believes one should train in cycles, beginning each cycle with a block of 12 to 16 weeks, then alternating the intensity and duration of the training. Wise participants schedule sufficient "days off," as the body needs this time for recovery. Following is the schedule favored by Dr. Anderson to enhance his power, endurance and flexibility.

MON.	TUE.	WED.	THU.	FRI.	SAT./SUN.
AM: Strength with weight training PM: Martial arts	AM: Aerobic cardiopulmonary bike or treadmill	DAY OFF	AM: Strength with weight training PM: Martial arts	AM: Aerobic cardiopulmonary bike or treadmill	Rest or Make-up Day if one day missed

It is inaccurate to define any form of exercise exclusively as aerobic or anaerobic, as variations of the activity may employ both forms of energy. We think of running as an excellent form of aerobic exercise. Yet, running can involve sprints (anaerobic). Weight training can involve high repetitions (100) with light resistance, thus recruiting aerobic and anaerobic benefits. What has been proven is that exercise in any form is rejuvenating, strengthening, and therapeutic. Men who include exercise as part of their life maintain a youthful elevation of testosterone levels later in life, while older men who have been inactive experience dramatic drops of testosterone levels, resulting in the acquisition of female characteristics, like pear-shaped bodies, higher and gentler voices, loss of facial and body hair, and generally delicate countenance. Part of this feminization is due to the natural fall of the hormone testosterone, as explained in our HRT chapter, but the process can be slowed by including anaerobic exercise in your daily regimen. Surprisingly, even aerobic exercise will increase testosterone levels 20% at the 20th minute of constant activity, 25% 10 minutes after exercise, and 21% 20 minutes after exercise, as reported in the *Journal of Strength and Conditioning Research*. The downside is that serum testosterone levels among these test subjects returned to baseline levels 30 minutes after aerobic exercise. Older life extensionists may have to boost their testosterone levels by ingesting precursors like DHEA and androstenedione. As a last resort, they can appeal to their complementary physician for injections of testosterone cypionate. Be sure to safeguard against prostate enlargement by including Saw Palmetto and Pygeum with any testosterone booster.

Obviously, in our quest for strong, active longevity, a balance of the two types of exercise, aerobic and anaerobic, is indicated. If you are really "out of shape" and have been inactive for a long time, take it easy. Start with just 20 minutes of walking. Check your pulse as described before and allow your pace to elevate your heart rate to 75% of maximum. (Remember, a good parameter for that measure is to subtract your age from the number 220 and multiply that number by .75). Keep up the pace and do not stop to smell the roses. (While we heartily believe in the appreciation of nature, take time for that on the way back). You'll feel stronger in a couple of weeks. Extend the time, then, striving for 30 minutes. Fat starts burning at the 16th minute, so you may want to stretch the aerobic duration longer if you have a plump problem, but don't go beyond an hour, no matter how fit or fat you feel, as prolonged aerobic exercise invites vast free radical damage. To protect against this offensive bombardment of oxidation, we take a minimum of 3 grams of Ester-C, 1200 units of Vitamin E, 50 mg of Tocotrienol, 50 mg of Grapeseed Extract, 200 mcg of Selenium, 30 mg CO Q-10, 100 mg of Alpha Lipoic Acid, and 25000 IU of Beta-Carotene, daily. All of these supplements are available over the counter.

After three months of such aerobic performance, you will have graduated from the "physically challenged" class. Congratulations! At that time, you should begin to insert intervals of sprinting into your 30-minute walk. These intervals may be as short as 30 seconds in duration, but do try to really sprint during that interval. For 3 weeks insert one 30-second sprint (alter the 16th minute of walking). Then, for the next 3 weeks, insert 2 fast intervals. After 3 more weeks, do three 30-second sprints. Work up to including 4 sprints during your 30-minute walk. This type of training is called high-intensity interval training, recommended years ago by Dr. Lawrence Morehouse, as mentioned in our *Muscles and Myths* segment, and more recently proposed by Shawn Phillips, an outstanding example of masculine physical development, who has revealed vital information in the cutting edge physical culture magazine, *Muscle Media 2000*, his brother Bill's publication. His marketing genius aside, Bill Phillips and his staff have contributed more to the science of natural physical development than anyone in the industry during these last years of the 20th century. A bodybuilder himself, who "dropped out" of the steroid society, Bill dared to expose the behemoth giants of championship bodybuilding as drug dependent pawns, supported by companies which produce bodybuilding supplements, major players in the world of economics as we approach the millennium. More important is his employment of a superb scientific staff responsible for bringing to the industry natural products like creatine, HMB, and Andro-6, to accelerate muscular development without drugs. We applaud

Bill, and other publishers who have taken his lead to rid the quest for the Perfect Form from drug dependency.

Results of a 1997 Creatine study by M. Englehardt, et al., confirm that a low dose of 6 grams per day increased the "interval power" of triathletes by 18%, so you might want to consider it, even at your early stage of exercise for the physically challenged.

R. Sharo, et al., at a 1998 San Francisco Experimental Biology Conference stated that with regard to damage prevention from catabolic processes, HMB is a forerunner of protective supplements (along with our recommended phosphatidyl serine). Since this study proved 50% less muscle damage among runners using 3 grams daily of thc supplement, and the same dosage has been reported by weight-resistance body builders to guard against catabolism caused by the stress of heavy duty exercise, it can be deduced that HMB is an effective protector against muscle damage from any prolonged physical effort.

Androstenedione, the principal ingredient of all "Andro" products, follows DHEA as a closer precursor to a male's production of his own testosterone, clarified in *Chapter Two* of this book. We feel compelled to recommend again that Saw Palmetto, Pygeum, and chrysin should be taken with any Andro product, to avoid prostate enlargement and aromatization that can cause the prohormone to take an estrogen pathway. Creatine, HMB, and Andro products are available over the counter at any reputable health product store or by mail order from ads in magazines like *Ironman*, *Muscle Magazine International*, and *Muscle Media 2000.* Of all the Andro products for men, 19-Norandrostenediol is the most effective, synergistic with 19-Norandrostenedione for optimum anabolic enhancement (with the least possible side effects that are undesirable). We advise women to take nothing stronger than DHEA, and no more than 25 mg daily.

DAY THREE

Torso time! While there are many exercises for torso development, we will focus upon one for rib cage expansion and two for chest and upper back muscular development.

Pullovers. The room for your vital organs is your rib cage. Some of you can see rib protrusions, stripped of your shirt; you are defined as ectomorphic. Some others, perhaps due to athletic involvement in your youth, have pectoral development that hides the upper ribs; you are called mesomorphic. The rest of you have fat drooping from your pectoral strands, resulting in enormous breasts, if you are female, and breast-like adipose tissue around the nipples if you are male; you are referred to as endomorphic. All of the above can benefit from the exercise called pullovers, designed for rib cage expansion, which the organs of your heart, lungs, and your liver will welcome, as they may be inordinately compressed. Teenagers can develop an enormous rib cage cavity, since the cartilage connecting their ribs to the sternum is still flexible.

With your feet on the floor and only the top of your back supported by the width of a bench, drop your butt lower than your chest. You will need a light weight to hold in your hands for optimum stretch; a Bible will do. You might consider reading a passage or two, while resting between sets. As you become more flexible, increase the weight to a large dictionary or perhaps a coffee table book about Leonardo da Vinci. After three months of this exercise, you will be ready to perform the same exercise with a small weight (pejoratively referred to as "dumbbells", a term, no doubt, coined by some feeble pencil neck who valued his intelligence). Frank's teenage son, Mark, shows good pullover form in Figure 136a. Inhale deeply as you slowly bring the weight behind your head with extended (but not locked) arms. Take 10 seconds to stretch back, 1 second to hold the extension, and 5 seconds to return to the start position. Drop your butt low as you reach the apogee of the movement, for maximum stretch. Do 3 sets of 10 reps.

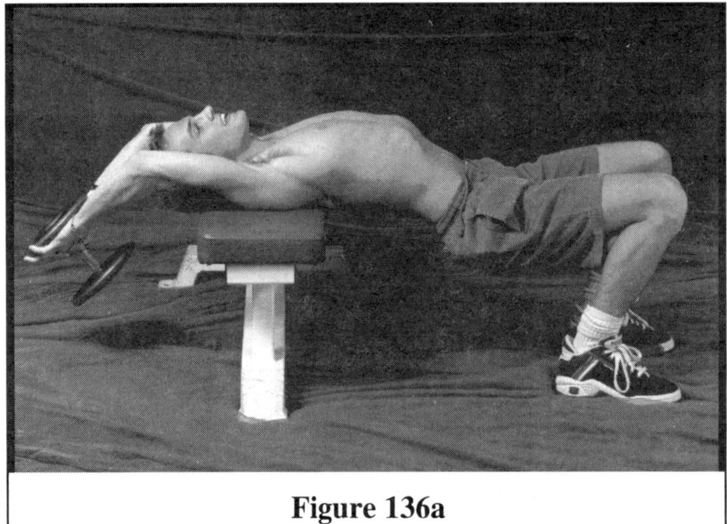

Figure 136a

Mark Covino incorporates pullovers into his workouts, which will eventually enlarge the rib cage and make more room for vital organs.

While pullovers are designed to open and stretch the rib cage, the return movement will develop the rib hugging serratus magnus muscles along with some fibers of the latissimus dorsi.

> Push-ups. Few readers are unfamiliar with this tortuous movement, used as a popular form of punishment by Army drill sergeants, but there is no better exercise for pectoral, deltoid and triceps development We can already hear some of you, the physically challenged, ranting, "I can't do that!"

The first step, in your quest for strong, active senior years is to remove the word can't from your vocabulary. You can, and, if you follow this simple approach, you will!

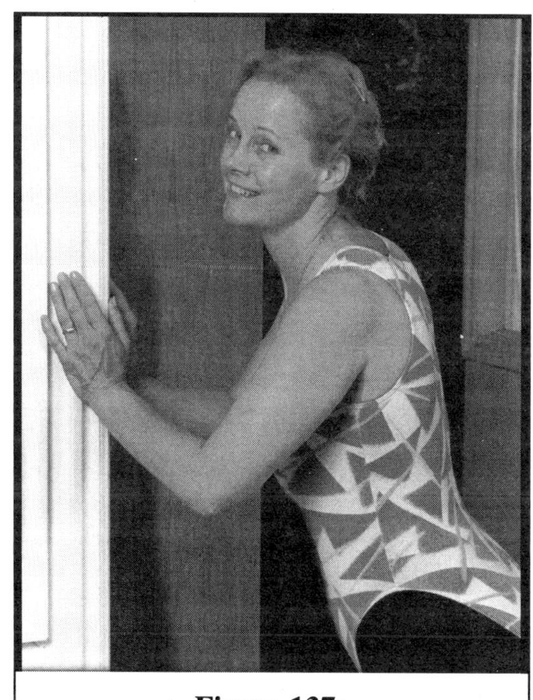

Figure 137a

Door jamb push-ups with slow repetitions can provide sufficient resistance for novice bodybuilders.

Begin by placing your hands upon an open door jamb at full arm's length. Bend your elbows, bringing your chest to the jamb, then slowly push back to the start position (Fig. 137a). Take 10 seconds to push back. Stop short of locking the elbows, hold for one second, tensing your pectorals and triceps, then take 5 seconds to return your chest to the door jamb. Do 3 sets of 10 reps.

If you find this too easy, you may not be as physically challenged as you think. You should try the same exercise with your hands on a table edge. When that becomes too easy, you're ready for the floor. Advanced body builders can have their partners rest on their back.

> Chin-ups. Before I admonish you for saying "can't" again, here is an approach that will soon have you proudly proclaiming, "I can!" Chin-ups will work the muscles that counter those involved in push-ups. Under stress will be the palmaris and biceps

of your arms, the broad latissimus dorsi of your back and the rhomboids of the upper back. With an overhand grip, your arms' brachialis and brachio-radialis muscles are summoned for further development.

Physically challenged readers should begin by lying on the floor with your head beneath a table. Reach up and grasp the table edge. Slowly pull up, taking 10 seconds to fully contract your biceps, hold for one second, tensing your upper arms, then take 5 seconds to lower to the start position. Perform 3 sets of 10 reps. If you cannot make 10, settle for 6 until you get stronger.

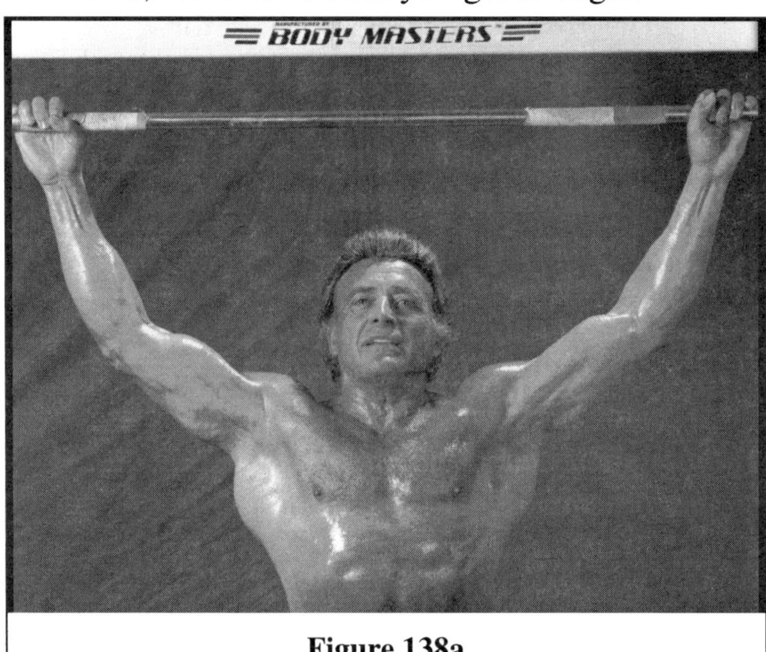

Figure 138a

Using a wide overhand grip during chin-ups enhances forearm development and stretches the latissimus dorsi muscles for a V-shaped silhouette.

From the floor, you will progress to a horizontal bar, as soon as you feel strong enough. If you are truly unable to perform a chin-up, try standing on a platform high enough to allow you to touch your feet to it when your arms are fully flexed, then buckle your knees to collapse them, until your arms are totally extended. Slowly pull your chin to the bar, as you begin your 10-1-5 cadence of seconds. When you can perform 3 sets of 10 reps (slowly), progress to 3 sets of 15 reps When you can accomplish 3 sets of 25, reps you will be ready for true chin-ups, with no problem. When you can perform 3 sets of 10 reps underhanded, consider the variation of gripping the bar overhanded. A wide grip will really stretch your back muscles (Fig. 138a). Advanced bodybuilders add a weight, suspended from a belt around their waist.

DAY FOUR

Waste the Waist. No amount of exercise, aerobic or anaerobic, will whittle the waist without proper dietary restrictions. Fat is fat, whether it is collected at your waist, as it is with most men, or is trapped in packets of cellulite hugging those saddlebags seen on many women. There are only two ways you can lose this weight. Either you burn more calories than you ingest or you become a fat-burning machine instead of a sugar-fired one.

The first method will certainly prevent more fat from accumulating, but this method will take a long time to show any evidence of old fat depletion. The second method enlists your own fat for energy, and, in the process of burning it, visible fat depletion will take place in two weeks. The obvious solution is to follow the second method first, until you have lost all visible signs of old adipose tissue, then, maintain your new silhouette by adopting the first method of ingesting fewer calories than you expend.

The second method is, of course, the ketogenic diet outlined by renowned cardiologist, Dr. Robert Atkins, and reviewed for you elsewhere in this book. Several days (more for some) after beginning a carbohydrate-free diet, you will enter a state of ketosis, wherein your brain, deprived of energy from sugar, will begin to attack your own fat, devouring it for energy. The change of your silhouette begins as early as the second week and dramatically continues. When you begin to replace complex carbs as advised, they will include vegetables, nuts and fruit that are low enough in carbohydrate content to not exceed your carb tolerance level (determined by Ketostix examination of your urine, as defined earlier).

Both methods for fat loss and maintenance will require booklets that list foods in order of carbohydrate content and caloric value; these can be found in any good book store and at the checkout counters of some supermarkets. Professional bodybuilders learn to limit their carbohydrate ingestion to less than 1 gram per pound of lean body weight, bumping their protein ingestion to 1.5 grams per pound of lean body weight and limiting their fat ingestion to 30% of all consumed food.

The major muscles that surround your waist include the rectus-abdominus set in the front, the spinal erectus which support the lumbar area of your spine, and the external oblique muscles at the sides. These muscles all can be developed with the same approach as is recommended for any muscle: Slow contraction and full extension, challenged by weight resistance sufficient to not permit an 11th repetition. For any muscular development, the augmentation of strength and size is directly related to the amount of time that a muscle is involved with tension against formidable resistance, so I personally have found the 10-1-5 cadence to be most effective. Follow every abdominal exercise with one for the spinal erectus or hyper-development of the former may shorten the abdominal muscles' length, making you less flexible. As we have advised, alternating exercises designed for antagonistic muscles will ensure flexibility plus strength. Yoga and other exercise modalities that feature stretching only do not develop phenomenal strength. Our goal is to develop a superhuman you.

> Crunches. So minimal is this movement, you will doubt its efficacy, but it truly works. The long rectus abdominus muscles are paired, running vertically from the base of the rib cage to the pubic area. They are corseted by three or four restrictive bands, adding great strength to the abdominal wall when the rectus abdominus is contracted. Dynamic tension during contraction will tear the muscle's fast twitch fibers. Hypertrophy will ensue during the recovery period, when dormant fibers are awakened and summoned to defend against the possibility of new stress. This is the basic science behind all muscular development. Crunches compress the rectus abdominus muscles, but continuous tension is necessary for their development.

Begin by pressing your back to the floor while you rest your feet on a bench, knees bent into a right angle. At first, place your hands on your upper stomach. When you get stronger, move your hands to your chest. Advanced bodybuilders hold a barbell plate on their chest for more resistance, on an inclined bench (Fig. 141a). Slowly raise your head and shoulders off the floor

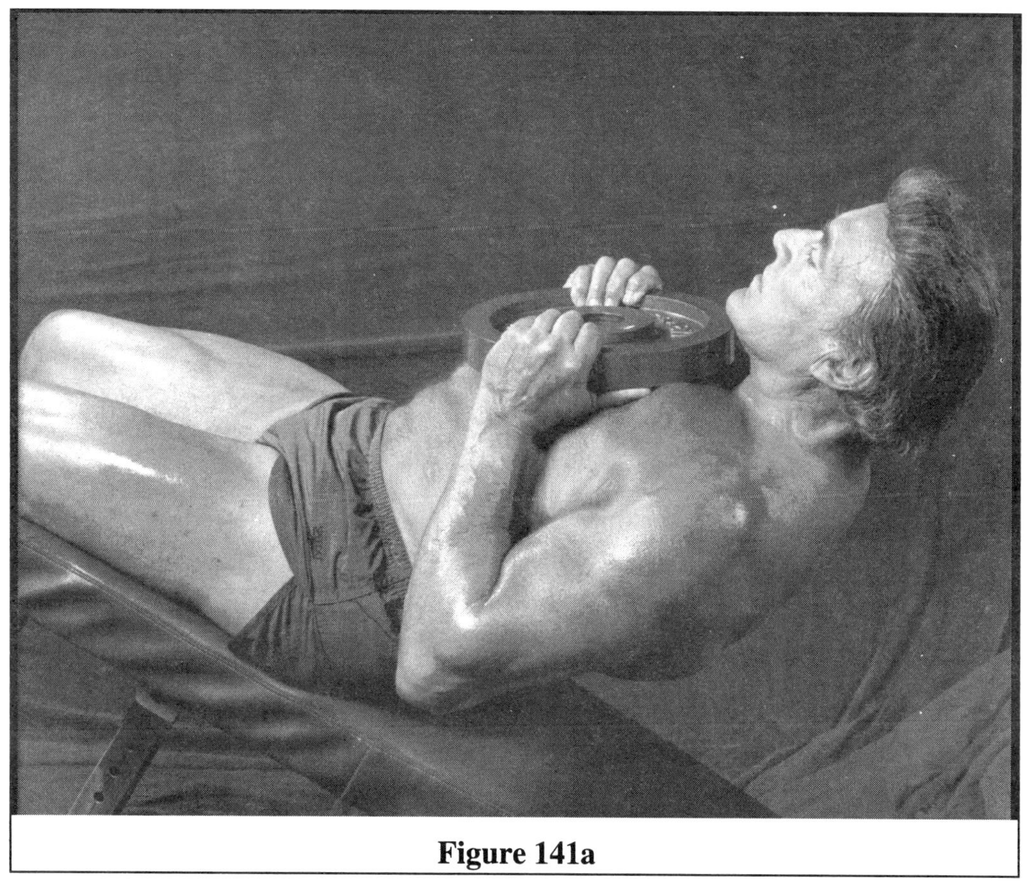

Figure 141a

Advanced crunches can be performed with a weight on top of the chest on an inclined bench.

or bench as you tense your abdominals. Take 10 seconds to rise to the position of full contraction. Hold and tense for a count of one, then take 5 seconds to return to the floor; 3 sets of 10 reps should be sufficient to promote upper abdominal wall development.

Reverse Crunches. For development below the navel, the movement can be reversed. Try it on a flat floor first. With your hands at your sides and your legs fully extended, bend your knees and bring them toward your chest, lifting your feet off the ground, slowly; 10 seconds to come up, hold the tension, squeezing your abdominals dynamically for one full second, then take 5 seconds to return. Try 3 sets of 10 reps. Dr. Anderson's wife, Amanda, shows good form in Figure 142a. Too tough? Give me 5 sets of 5 reps until you get stronger. Advanced bodybuilders keep their legs straight, graduating to an inclined board for more resistance and its resultant stress.

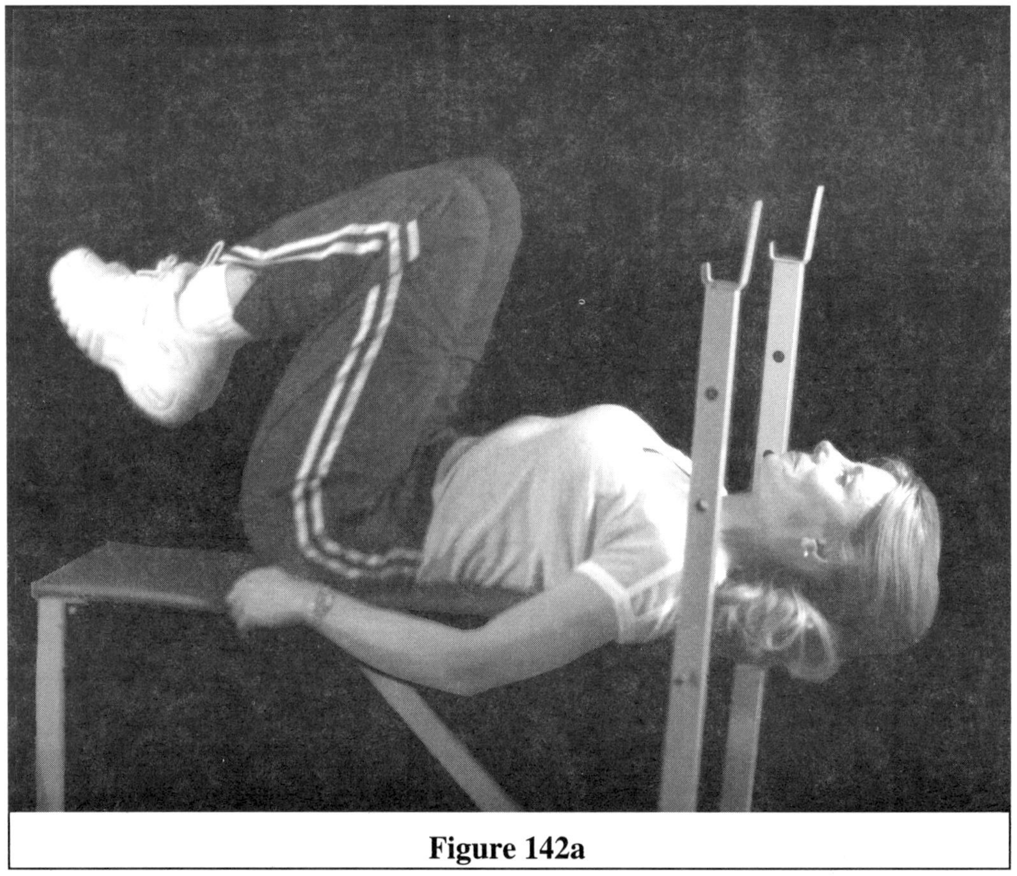

Figure 142a

Amanda Anderson performs a reverse crunch on a straight bench, raising bent knees toward her chest.

Ohio Gozaimus. This phrase means "good morning" in Japanese and is usually accompanied by a bow of the torso from the waist. Our Oriental friends must have well-developed spinal erectus muscles, the principal power center for this humble movement. Performed slowly, to the 10-1-5 cadence specified before, physically challenged bodybuilders should need no extra resistance. Take a wide stance with your hands on your hips, at first. When you get stronger, try the bow with your hands behind your head. Bow forward until your torso is parallel to the ground (Fig. 143a). Advanced bodybuilders perform this lower back developing exercise with a barbell behind their necks.

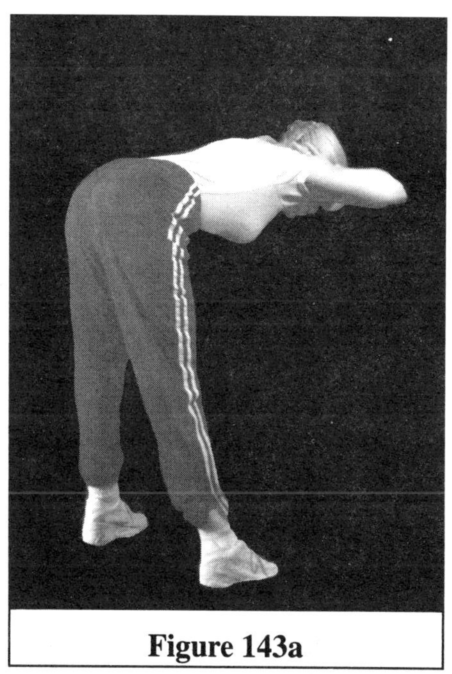

Figure 143a

The Ohio Goziamus or "good morning" exercise strengthens the lower back.

Flatten the Tire. If your external obliques are hidden by the clone of an inner tube, you must consider these side-bends, although this area-specific exercise will be a fruitless effort without a proper diet. A heavy book once again can provide sufficient resistance until you get strong enough to use a dumbbell.

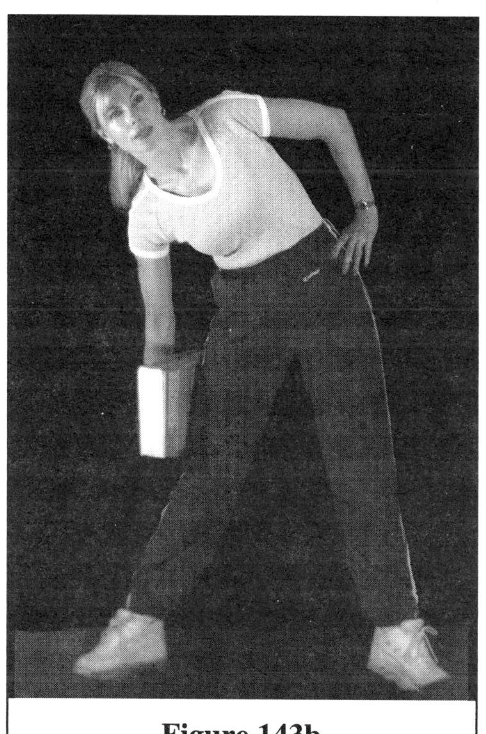

Figure 143b

Get rid of your "love handles" with side bends.

Stand with your feet shoulder-width apart, holding your book in one hand. Slowly drop the book to knee level; this is your starting position. You will feel a stretch or pull of your external oblique on the working side that is opposite the book (Fig. 143b). Take 10 seconds to raise to an erect posture, tense the working muscle for a count of one, then take 5 seconds to return to your starting position. Your goal is 3 sets of 10 reps for each side. Start with less reps if you are weak in this area.

Day Four is done. Get some rest and do not cheat on your diet. Tomorrow is another aerobic day.

DAY FIVE

Employ the same aerobic schedule you followed on Day Two. It is, of course, best if you can walk/run outdoors (never in an auto-polluted environment, though). For those of you who live in a crowded city, there is that wonderful machine called a treadmill. If I must resort to a treadmill while on the road, I set the pace at 3 with a high elevation of 15 and catch up on my reading, interrupting the pace 4 times with sprints at a speed level of 7. A high elevation will simulate hill walking, much safer and more beneficial, as the knee remains flexed, avoiding compression damage, and the soleus muscle will be more thoroughly stretched. All health clubs offer a variety of designs for the treadmill, which has become a most popular machine.

DAY SIX

Quads day. There are three major muscles on the front of your leg and one split set on the back, mirroring the construction of your arms. Front and center is your rectus femoris, flanked by the tear-drop shaped vastus internus on the inside of the thigh and the vastus externus sweeping down the side. Behind the thigh are the contraction muscles, know as the biceps femorus and the semitendinosus. We need to stress them all, for optimum thigh development, including the strap-like sartorius, longest of all the leg muscles, on the inside of your thigh If you still have the stamina, we will also work out the lower leg muscles during this exercise period.

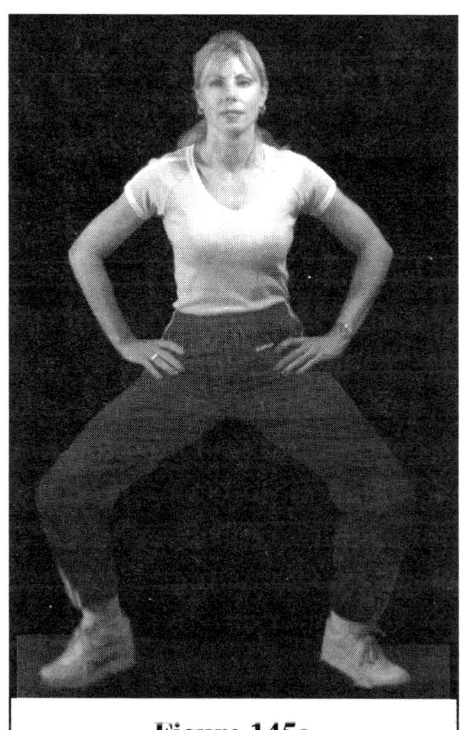

Figure 145a

Slow, wide-stance pliés provide sufficient stress for leg muscles, especially quadriceps.

Wide Stance Plié. Spread your feet a bit wider than your shoulders, and point them away from each other. With your hands on your hips, slowly descend into a "squat," until your thighs are parallel to the floor. Stop; this is your starting position. Take 10 seconds to rise. Hold the contraction just before knee lock-out and squeeze the thigh muscles with forceful tension. Try for 3 sets of 10 reps; less reps and more sets if you are weaker (Fig. 145a).

Leg Curls. For optimum thigh development and protection of the anterior cruciate ligament of the knee, try these with the help of a friend. Figure 145b shows the apogee or moment of dynamic tension. Take 10 slow seconds to get there. Hold for a hard squeeze count of one. Take 5 seconds to return. Your partner can offer pull resistance for your contraction and push resistance for your return.

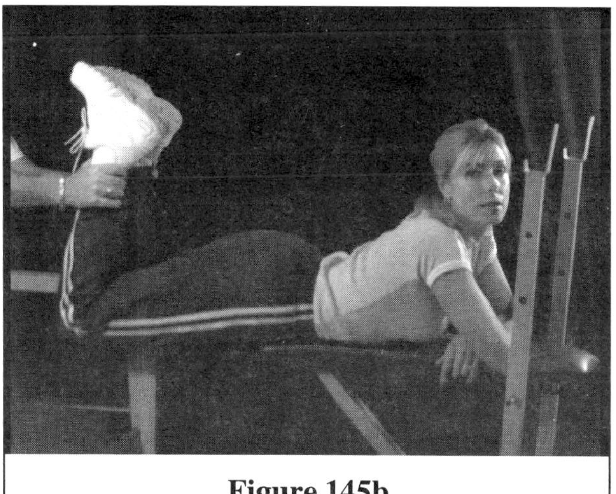

Figure 145b

Dr. Anderson provides resistance for his wife's leg curls. Fully contracted, Amanda will hold the tension for a count or two before returning to start position.

Toe Raises. Your calves are probably the most difficult muscle to develop, since you use them for walking every day. The medical term for this important muscle is gastrocnemius. To contract it, you must rise up on your toes. For full extension, try toe raises on a thick book (Fig. 146a), which will permit your heels to lower. For added resistance, try one-legged toe raises. Advanced bodybuilders use resistance machines. Before you reach that point, try the leg raises one-legged, seated, with your partner sitting on your knee. Remember to rise slowly, taking 10 seconds to fully contract; squeeze a tense count of one second; then lower your heel during a 5 count. Your calves should burn when you have completed 3 sets of 10.

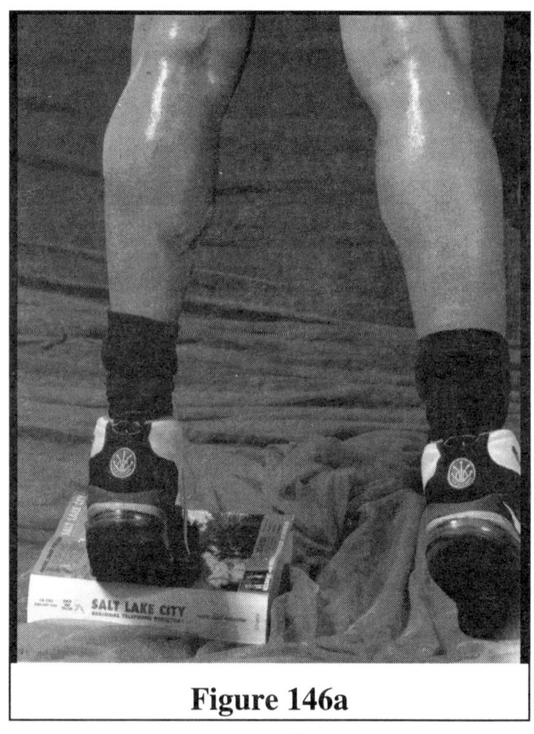

Figure 146a

Try toe raises on a thick book for a full extension.

DAY SEVEN

On the seventh day your Creator rested, and certainly, you should, too. Try for a physically stress-free day. Complete relaxation. If your diet has been strict and you feel deprived, enjoy something you miss most. Yes, even that chocolate sundae with whipped cream, or pizza with a mug of Guinness, all with one condition: Before you pig out on carbohydrates, ingest some kind of protein, even if it must be supplemental, as in the form of ten desiccated liver capsules. Attend your house of worship, eat and take a nap; watch a movie, but avoid anything that produces physical stress. Read. Meditate. Pray. Tomorrow, repeat the week's schedule we have recommended. Continue this program until you feel you are ready for exercise with weight resistance (the only form of exercise that has been proven to develop lean tissue and sculpt your body to a silhouette that you were designed to have) training with weight resistance is the corner stone on the Fountain of Youth !

Weight Resistance Exercise to Combat the Agonizing Atrophy of Aging

Like many clichés, the adage, "What you don't use, you lose," rings true with regard to the muscles you were given to sustain the physical demands of human life. Our Creator blessed us with a brain capable of extraordinary intellectual achievement and a skeleton supported by muscle capable of incredible feats of strength, but if the brain is not educated and not nourished by nutrients transported through the blood stream, it will waste, shrivel, and die long before its programmed life span, and so will the body's muscle. Brain and muscle atrophy are the principal players in the drama of early mortality. Hormones were designed to decline gradually after the first quarter of a century with little remaining during the last quarter. Complementary physicians have countered this natural aging development with hormone replacement therapy, predicting extemporization of this practice to be a primary thrust of 21st-century-medicine, in its effort to prolong active longevity. But research offers evidence that the brain and the muscles of our bodies are not predestined to deteriorate at any milestone of age, as both can be nourished and stimulated to grow at any time during the human life span. This evidence suggests that maximum strength and intellectual achievement need not require the compulsory prerequisite of youth. Men and woman of "retirement age" are less mentally alert and weaker than the younger generation of their time because of a self-adopted pattern of lethargy, not by natural design. Your debilitation is self-inflicted, not inherited. You have chosen to retire your brain after your school days and chosen to move slower, placing less demand upon your muscle, because you have conned yourself into believing that you should "act your age" or that mental and physical achievement are the exclusive activities of the young and beautiful. Hogwash!

Because education requires mental effort with extensive research and strength requires physical resistance against formidable forces, some choose to avoid both as adults, as though maturity awards them license for lethargy, hedonism, and recalcitrance. Many adults revert to the status of pre-school children, gleefully stuffing their expanding guts with all forms of the sugar we felt deprived of as children, retiring to the couch (in place of the crib) to be fed and entertained by others. Why read, when we can watch TV? Why be physically active when we can pay young athletes outrageous salaries to play games we can watch? Why create art, when we can plaster our walls with cheap prints?

This process of self-inflicted aging often begins with marriage. Until that time, we sense that mental and physical development are necessary to offer a countenance that will attract potential mates. The 50% current divorce rate may be partly explained by the relaxation of both interests, once the ceremony ends, and particularly after the first child is born. The world then begins to revolve around baby. Postpartum blues are precursors to sexual avoidance and eventual repulsion, as Mommy becomes matronly and Daddy begins to allow blubber to hang over his belt. Driving us deeper into the comfort of the couch, replete with TV clicker, is the sigh, "What a relief. I don't have to look physically attractive anymore, I'm married," or, "I'm a mom" or, "I'm a dad." Health club registers list vast numbers of divorced members, reluctantly in repair to ameliorate body distortions that resulted from the seductive security of marriage. Their renewed interest in physical development is motivated by the mating game. Again, many health clubs are replacing the smoke-filled singles bars for the mating ritual. Whatever the motivation, the primary lesson to be learned from this amusing cultural development is that the body at any age will respond to physical stress with hypertrophy of muscle and athletic endurance, if the stress is periodic, progressively demanding, and if the body is fueled with proper nourishment during the bodybuilding process.

For dramatic resculpting of the human form, only one form of exercise never fails: It involves no game; there are no scores to keep; and you are not called upon to "hit or conquer." This exercise can, however, be classified as a form of self-defense, as the resultant strength and endurance that follows dedicated participation will prepare you for any sport or physically demanding activity, and participation may prolong your life. The exercise should be identified with the label "bodybuilding." The physical stress and resultant muscular development is induced by weight resistance. Although it involves the lifting of weights, we avoid the label weight<u>lifting</u>, reserving that for the competitive hoisting of incredible poundages. The world's "strongest" men today may be impressed with their power, but most have incredibly fat bellies that jiggle and vie with their chests for girth, far from being healthy physical specimens. The bodybuilder's quest is for symmetry, a classical form, strength, and good health.

Weight resistance against human effort places stress upon corresponding muscle. If the stress is sufficient, the muscle affected by it will tear. During the resting phase, catabolism of the stressed muscle will result if it is not fed proper nutrients to support repair. Nutrients like protein, glutamine, complex carbohydrates and creatine, fed to the stressed muscle, will bring it repair and added strength; the process also feeds dormant muscle fibers, which are recruited to guard against more stress in the future. Repeated stress, i.e., a regular regimen of exercise will stimulate the pituitary gland to secrete Growth Hormone, raising IGF-1 levels (insulin growth factor), a potent anabolic (muscle-building) hormone; testosterone levels will also rise in men and women, giving a boost to the muscle nutrients, and the result of all this stimulation and fuel is more strength. If the movement and its resistant weight is frequent and light, i.e., high repetitions with low weight, strength and endurance will ensure. If the weight resistance is high and the movement is slow, i.e., low, slow repetitions with heavy weight, strength and noticeable hypertrophy of the stressed muscle will follow. Since an exercise exists for every muscular area of your body, you can thus sculpt any shape you desire. While spot reduction may not be possible (without surgery), spot development is achievable with weight-resistance exercise. (It should be noted that recent supplementation of the male prohormone DHEA by women bodybuilders has challenged this spot-reduction premise, since many are reporting significant depletion of fat in the hips and thighs due to their androgenic response to this natural supplement).

There is no doubt, however, that weight-resistance exercise can spot-develop. Women respond to weight resistance twice as fast as men, as reported in *Health Magazine*, 1998. As we have explained, strength and muscular development takes place during the recuperative phase and not during the time of exercise, when the muscle is literally torn. For this reason, sufficient rest must follow every weight-resistance encounter. Wise bodybuilders exercise a different body part each exercise session, allowing for plenty of muscle recuperation and regeneration between stressful encounters; this also gets you out of the gym quicker. One hour should be sufficient time for you to exercise one or two body parts. The following exercises comprise your author's current regimen. As we have specified, we will not prescribe, but should you decide to follow this course for three months and not see dramatic progress in your health and physical countenance, you may trash our book and we will give you your old body back!

ARMS DAY

Arms can take a lot of punishment, and since they are involved with all other torso exercises, my preferred schedule is to work them hard on the first day, work my legs on day two, perform cardio and stomach work on the third day, work upper back and shoulders on day four, chest and lower back on day five, and rest and recuperate on the weekends. The body responds well to variety, though, so I change the routine every few months. For size and strength, I keep carbohydrates under 50 mg during the week with no limit on the weekends, but try to ingest 1 gram of protein for every pound of my body weight every day. To lose weight when I carried too much fat, I enlisted ketone energy by limiting my carbs to under 35 mg every day. The body fat depleted, but my arms and other muscles did not achieve much size and I felt tired. The anabolic variation of diet described first gives me the size and energy I prefer. The diet was borrowed from bodybuilding guru Dan Duchaine, revealed in his excellent book *Body Opus*. Here is the routine I follow on Arms Day:

Warm-up. Many bodybuilders avoid the warm-up, because it involves very light-weight and high repetitions. It is an ego thing. (Suppose somebody sees us!) What the warm-up does is awaken the scheduled muscles to prepare them for high stress. To avoid the warm-up is to invite pain and cramping the following day. Since the arms are our target this first day, a composite warm-up exercise that involves the arms will work best. One of the best exercises is the alternate curl and press, using a very light dumbbell in each hand; the poundage should be sufficient to not permit a 26th repetition.; this, of course, will differ between every individual. You must determine the amount. Try a set with a light weight. If this weight permits more than 25 repetitions, rest, then try another set with dumbbell that is 5 lbs. heavier. You will have to do a lot of experimenting on this first day to determine your specific exercise poundages.

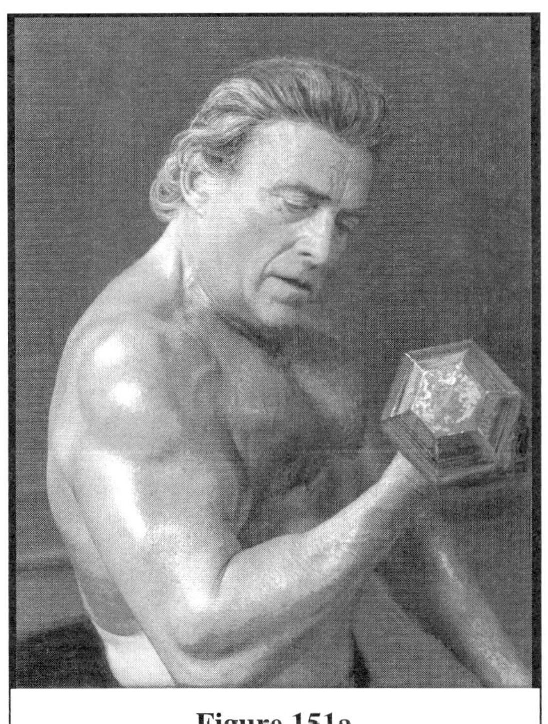

Figure 151a

Slowly curl the weight upward, turning your fist until the back of your hand faces forward.

Hold the dumbbells at your side, with your knuckles and fingertips against your thighs. If the gym has a bench with a short back rest, you will put less stress upon your back and sacroiliac.

Slowly curl the left dumbbell to your shoulder, without moving your elbow. As you curl it up, turn your fist until the back of your hand faces forward (Fig. 151a). Then, press the dumbbell overhead, twisting your hand again to end with the palm of your hand facing forward (Fig. 151b).

This compound movement is considered to be one repetition. As you lower the dumbbell reversing the movement described, curl and press the other dumbbell in the same manner. Try for 25 reps with each arm; if you find that difficult, use less weight. Rest for a minute or two and begin the next exercise.

Biceps Curls. The biceps is the long muscle on the front of the arm which swells to a globe when it is flexed Any movement of your hand to full arm extension to your shoulder is called a curl. All types of curls place stress upon the biceps. There are many variations, and the use of one or two arms is optional. Two-arm exercises are faster, but if time is not a critical concern, one-arm exercises isolate the muscle under stress for concentrated focus and resultant hypertrophy. Figure 152a shows a one-arm variation, using a cable machine. Figure 152b shows a two-arm curl on a "Scott" bench, named

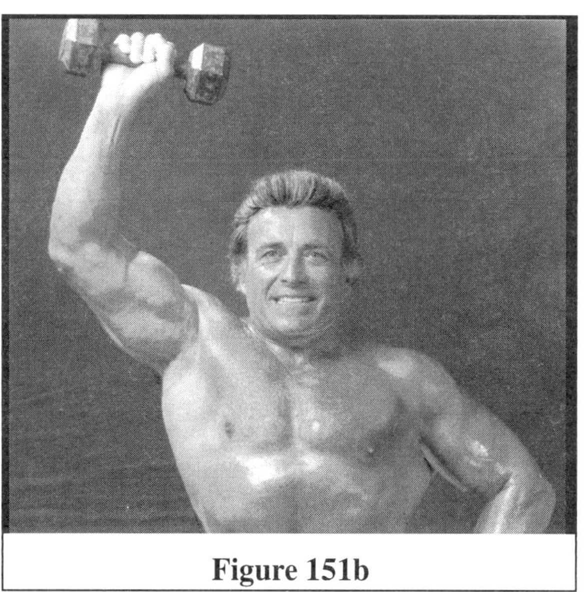

Figure 151b

As you press the weight overhead, end with the palm of your hand forward.

after its inventor who provided the device to further isolate the biceps muscle, using the elbow as a fulcrum. For this and most of the muscle-building exercises in my schedule, I prefer a 10-1-5 cadence, 10 seconds to curl or contract, one second to hold and tense the targeted muscles, and 5 seconds to lower the weight back to full arm extension. This slow cadence produces more time under tension, proven to stress the working muscle with maximum intensity.

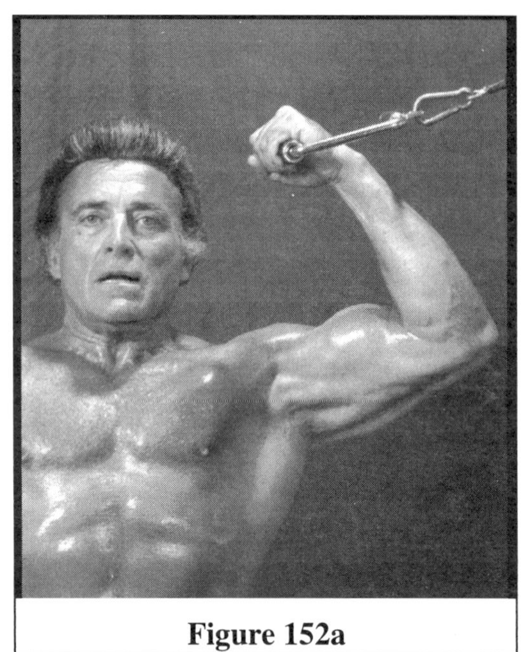

Figure 152a

A one-arm variation of the Bicep Curl using a cable machine.

For repetitions, I prefer 10 for the first set (an 11th should be impossible), 8 for the second set, and 6 for the final set, increasing the poundage for each set to guarantee failure beyond the prescribed number of reps. Be sure to rest for no more than 3 minutes between each set. If you perform curls one arm at a time, follow the first set of 10 reps by switching immediately to the other arm. While this arm is working, the other will be resting and should have recuperated sufficiently for another set when the exercises for the second arm are completed. Aerobic exercise is oxygen-driven, constant and relentless. Anaerobic exercise is driven by muscle and fat energy used against formidable resistance. No rest between exercises can produce aerobic <u>and</u> anaerobic benefits. Moreover, such a routine will call upon Type 1 and Type 2 fibers for total muscular development. These fibers are frequently labeled fast twitch and slow twitch, the former responding to heavy weight resistance and the latter called upon for long bouts of endurance. With little rest throughout the routine you should feel oxygen-deprived. Breathe in deeply and blow out your carbon

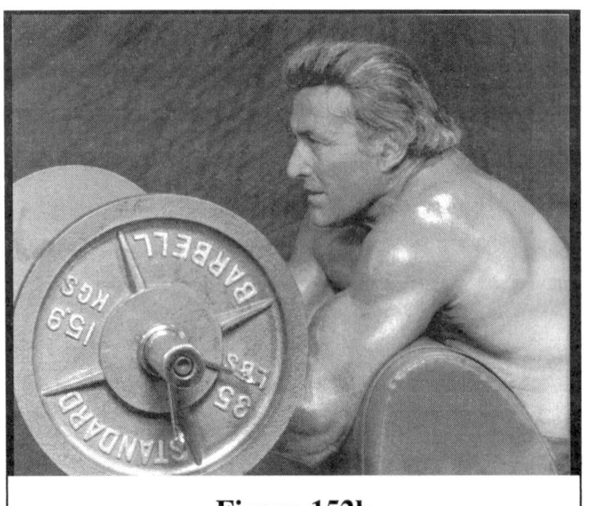

Figure 152b

A two-arm Bicep Curl using a Scott bench.

dioxide forcibly during and after the exercise. Drink at least 10 gulps of water.

Contraction exercise followed by extension movements can protect against the shortening or binding of a muscle, The body is constructed with systems of what artists call contrapunta (counterpoint); for every force there is a complementary opposing force. For every muscle that effects contraction, there is an opposing muscle that is provided for extension. If both areas are not stressed and developed, the working muscle may shorten and bind. The "muscle-bound" image of some bodybuilders is due to their lack of attention to antagonistic muscles designed to provide a flexible balance. Curls alone could develop massive biceps on the front of the upper arm, but with equal time not given to the triceps group on the back of thc uppcr arm, the biceps range could shorten, preventing full arm extension. Stone sculptors often develop such a bind in their hammer driving arm. To prevent such binding, I like to follow contraction exercises for the biceps with extension exercises that stress the triceps group.

Triceps Extensions. Often called French Curls, this movement can be performed with one or two arms, developing the three muscles that hug the

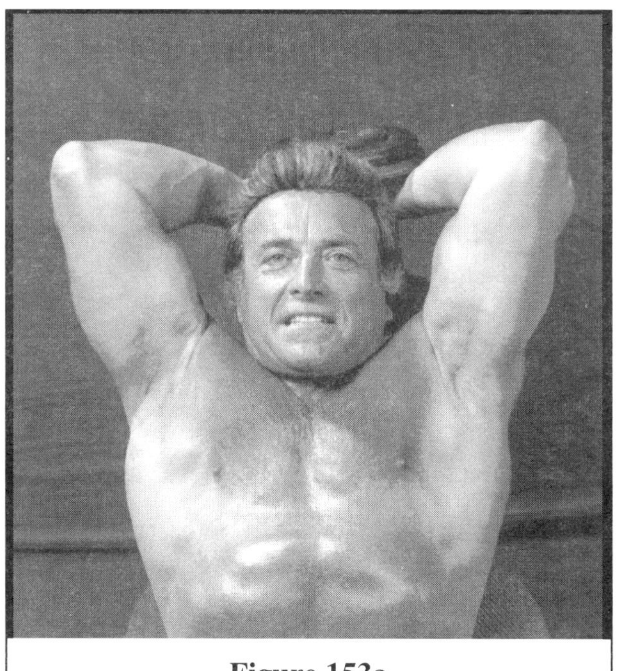

Figure 153a

A two-arm variation of the "French" Curl. Start with elbows close to your ears.

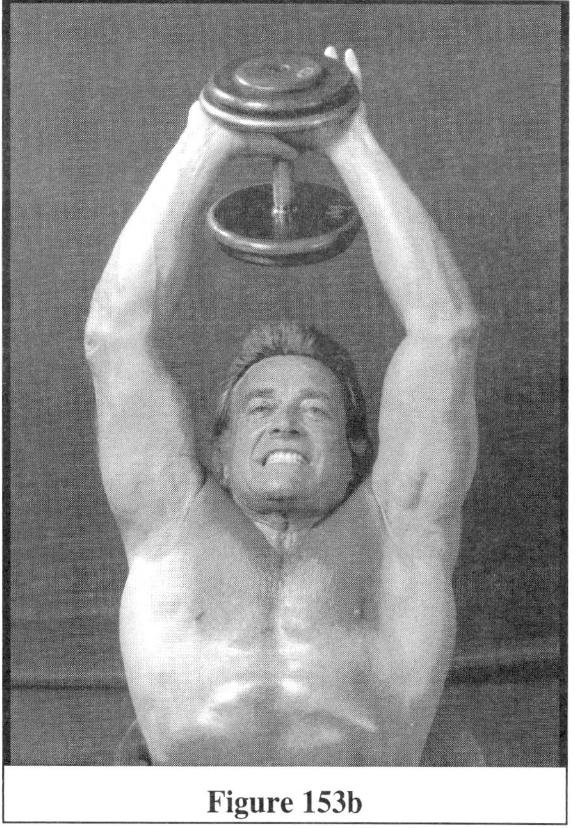

Figure 153b

Extend fully with elbows stationary.

back of the arm; the triceps is shaped like a horseshoe. The exercise can be performed while reclining on a bench or while sitting on a bench with a low back rest. Figure 153a shows the seated two-arm variation. The elbow functions as a fulcrum from the flexed position to full arm extension over the head (Fig. 153b). After a warm-up set with a light weight, increase the poundage to allow 10 repetitions. Press slowly, taking 10 seconds to extend the arm, one second to tense the triceps and 5 seconds to descend back to the starting position. Use a weight that will demand failure after ten repetitions for the first set, 8 reps for set two, and 6 reps for the final set; this is called "working to failure." Once the last prescribed repetition becomes easy enough to permit another rep, you are advised to increase the poundage. Drink.

Hammer Curls. Between the biceps and triceps is a contracting muscle that curls the arm upward from full extension when the hand faces the thigh, called the brachialis. The movement resembles that which is called upon to hammer a nail or chisel, hence the name (Fig. 154a). I occasionally perform this exercise on an inclined bench for greater extension. Development of the brachialis is essential for full arm size, and there is no better exercise for its isolation than the Hammer Curl, preferably performed one arm at a time.

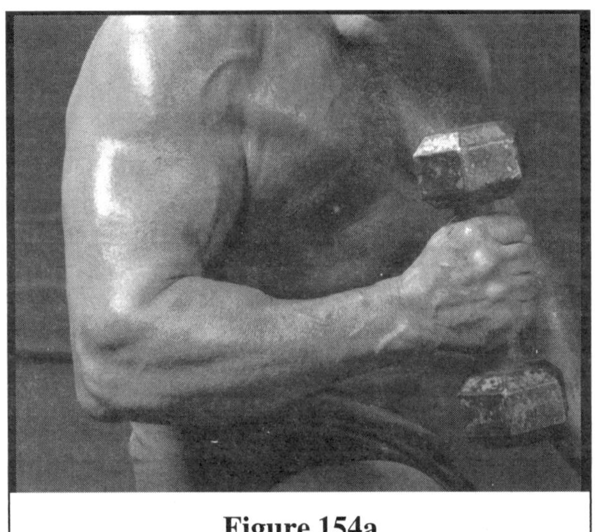

Figure 154a

Perform Hammer Curls slowly.

After the customary 25 reps with a light weight for warm-up, 3 sets with sufficient weight increase to perform 10 reps, 8 reps, and a final 6 reps to failure will surely stress this vital muscle. From a full-arm extension, curl the weight up slowly, 10 seconds to come up, one second to hold and squeeze the contraction, and 5 seconds to lower. Continue, alternating arms. Drink.

Upright Triceps Extensions. Figure 155a shows the two-arm press down, requiring a triceps extension machine, found in any good health club, These presses are performed while standing, with the elbows stationary, following the same 10-1-5 cadence, increasing resistance poundage with each set, to accommodate 10 reps, 8 reps, and a final 6 reps, all, of course, to failure, Figure 155b shows the one-arm variation. Notice the reverse grip, and the inverted horseshoe shape of my triceps. Allow the hand to press down the weight without moving the elbow for total triceps isolation. Your upper arms should be swollen from cell volumization by now. The tight feeling is referred to by professional bodybuilders as the rush of being "pumped," but you are not done, yet. Drink.

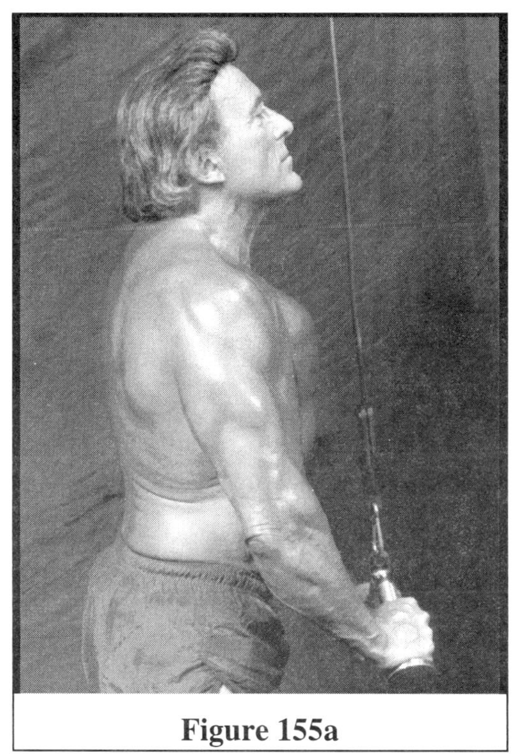

Figure 155a

Keep elbows stationary and movement slow during two-arm Tricep Press Downs.

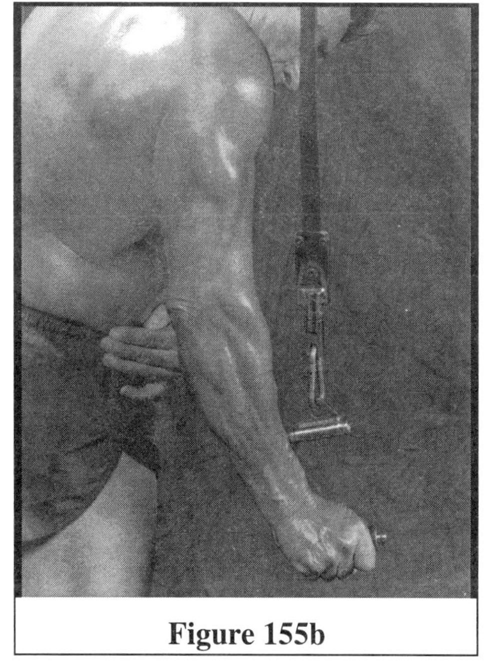

Figure 155b

One-arm variation of Tricep Press Down. The elbows must not move.

Palmaris Wrist Curls. Although the forearms are partially involved while performing the first ten exercises, an isolated movement will keep the girth of the forearm in symmetrical balance with the upper arm when hypertrophy of the latter ensues. There is no better movement for development of the palmaris than the one-arm Wrist Curl.

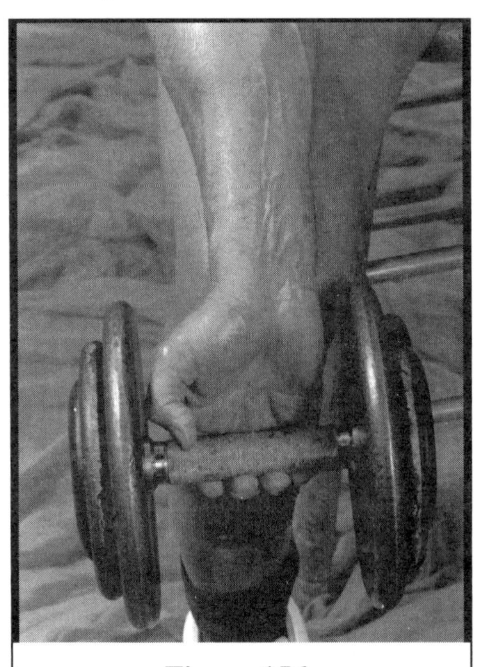

Figure 156a

Wrist Curl start position. Let the bar drop to your fingertips.

Sit on a bench, resting the back of your forearm on one thigh. Allow the bar of your chosen weight to drop to a fingertip grip (Fig. 156a). Slowly curl the weight upward, using only your fingertips. Take 5 seconds to curl, hold, and squeeze the palmaris for a count of one (Fig. 156b), then take 5 seconds to roll back to the starting position. Three sets of graduated weight increase to permit failure after 10 reps, 8 reps, and then 6 reps should swell the palmaris and make it burn. Alternate your arms, so that one forearm rests while the other is working. Drink.

Your arms should feel pumped. Your arm day workout is complete. You can expect some pain the next day. This afterburn is felt two days later by your author, perhaps because of my age. The afterburn accounts for the cliché: "No pain, no gain," originally used to describe ineffective workouts, where the bodybuilder did not push himself to failure. Part of the pain may be due to lactic acid accumulation, but more likely, it accompanies repair of torn muscle tissue, which takes place between workouts when the torn muscle is in repair. Extra magnesium supplementation after each workout can help lessen the pain of torn tissue. The antioxidants N-acete-cystine, Pycnogenol,

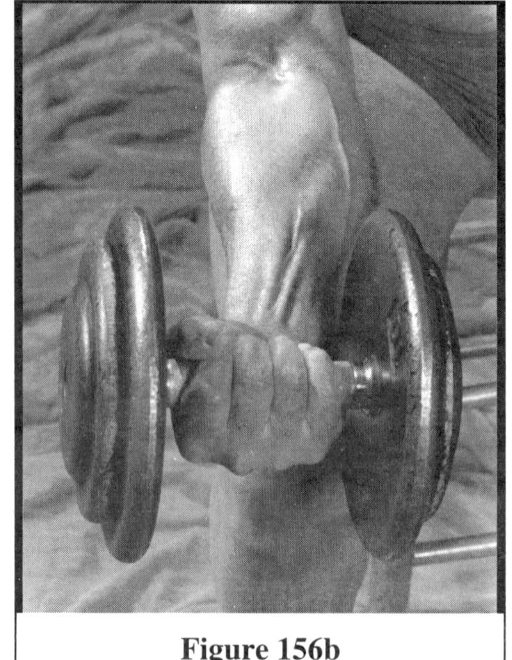

Figure 156b

The finish position of the Wrist Curl contracts the Palmaris.

vitamin E and vitamin C will guard against free radical invasion that usually accompanies post-workout pain. Phosphatidyl serine (about 400 mg) and 3 grams of HMB daily will guard against cortisol secretion and resultant catabolism, while 2 grams of glutamine supplementation 3 to 5 times a day will ensure growth of new muscle tissue along with repair of the damaged fibers. You have about a two-hour window after high-intensity muscle stress to pop in those supplements and avoid discouraging catabolism. Chase these supplements down with a high-protein, high-carb drink to replenish your expended glycogen and encourage protein synthesis. Add a 5-gram scoop of creatine to the drink. Drink plenty of water.

LEG DAY

Your arms will welcome at least two days of rest after stressing them with high intensity. I like to follow arm day with a leg workout and follow that day with cardio and abdominals work, to give the arms total rest. During the two torso days that end my week, the arms are partially activated, but the arm day workout just defined is not repeated for another week.

Since the knees are critical joints, necessarily stressed with all weight-resistance leg work, it is important to begin their activation with a high-repetition, low-weight warm-up. Best for this exercise is a combination of leg extensions and leg curls, alternated with 25 reps each. Follow with 3 sets of high-intensity, heavy-resistance movements, like squats or leg presses, utilizing the 10-1-5 cadence and increasing the weight resistance for each set. Leg extensions stress the anterior muscles of the thigh, while leg curls work the posterior leg biceps.

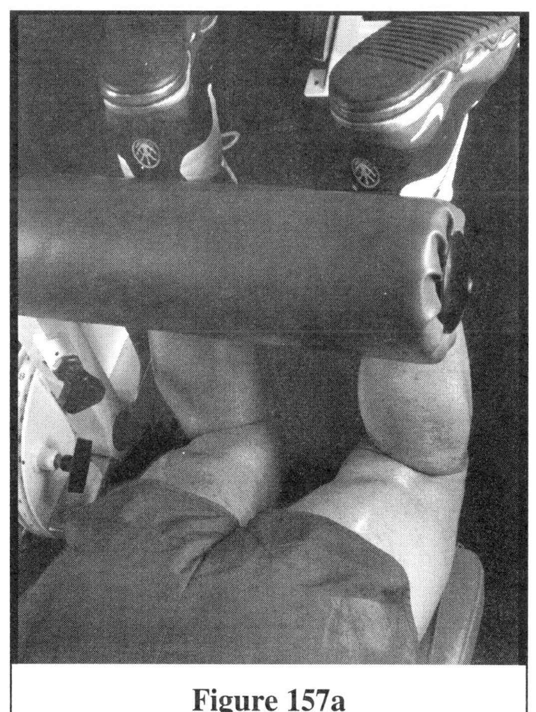

Figure 157a

Fully contracted Leg Curl. Hold the tension for a count or two before returning to the start position.

Leg Curls. You will find a leg curl machine at every reputable health club, usually positioned next to the leg extension machine, since they know you will probably want to mix a contraction exercise with an extension movement to ensure flexibility. Dr. Anderson and his wife have their own apparatus in their home gym.

Stretch out on the bench face down, hooking your Achilles tendons under the padded roll bar. Set the poundage pin into a light weight that will permit 25 reps and begin your warm-up set of leg curls (Fig. 157a). Rest a minute while you change the pin to a weight that will permit 10 reps to failure. Perform them with a 10-1-5 cadence and rest. Increase the weight to an eight rep limit for the next set. Increase the weight again for a maximum of six repetitions. Drink.

Leg Extensions. The 3 muscles that front the thigh are similar to the triceps of your upper arm and are also used for extension. The leg extension exercise can follow your 3 sets of leg curls, or, you might prefer to alternate contractions with extensions, as I do: A set of 10 leg curls followed by a set of 10 leg extensions, with no rest in between. I move on quickly to a set of 8 leg curls followed by 8 leg extensions, and finish with a set of 6 leg curls followed by 6 leg extensions, each set increasing the weight to work to failure. With no rest between exercises, some aerobic benefit will surely accompany the anaerobic activity. Your knees will be well juiced for the heavy resistance that will follow.

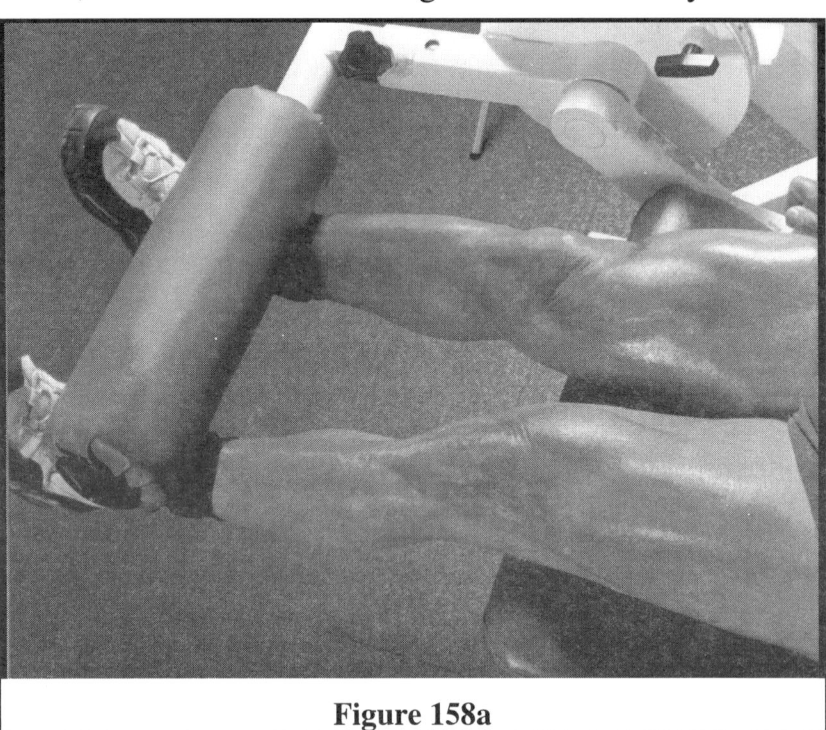

Figure 158a

Leg extensions develop the quadriceps of the thighs. Hold the contraction for a count or two before lowering the weight to start position.

Begin leg extensions by sitting on the bench with your insteps hooked under the padded roll bar. Slowly raise the weight with a 10-1-5 cadence. Squeeze the contraction of the anterior leg muscles for a count of one second just before lockout (Fig. 158a). Avoid total locking of the knee joint as this can be stressful to the patella. Point the toes straight ahead for rectus femoris emphasis. Point the toes inward to place more emphasis upon the vastus externus and outward for vastus internus concentration. With these varied approaches, you can sculpt your own thighs. Rest no more than 3 minutes between exercises. Drink.

Leg Presses. Leg presses may be substituted for leg "squats", if you are older, as the latter exercise stresses the vertebrae dangerously from

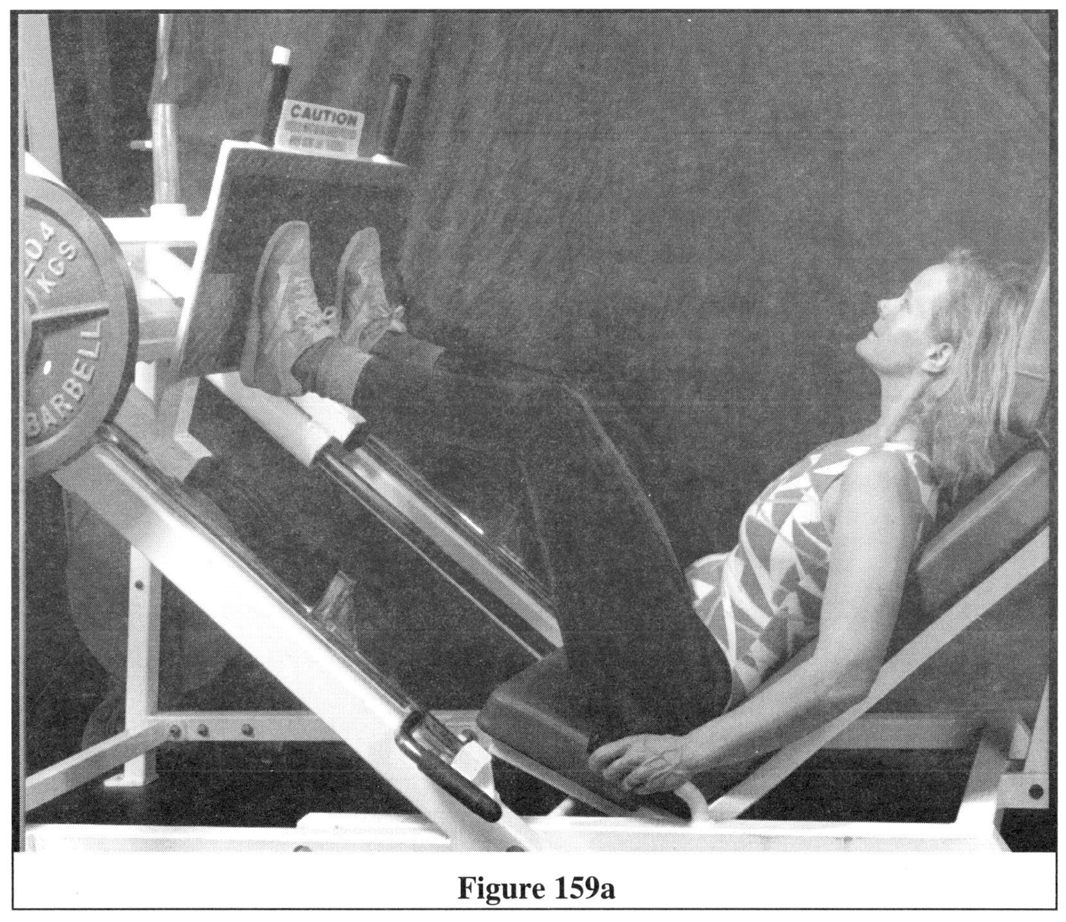

Figure 159a

Vary the space between feet during leg presses for total thigh development. Lower weight until lower legs are at right angle to thighs, then immediately press weight upward.

compression, and older bones are usually more brittle. Curiously, weight-resistance exercise will promote bone density, especially if the exercise is begun during the high-testosterone years. Vermont osteopathic surgeon, Dr. Robert Johnson remarked that your retirement age author's x-rays show the bone density of an athletic 30-year-old. Participants of all ages are advised to include calcium supplementation along with their multiple vitamin and mineral capsules for bone protection. Women, prone to osteoporosis in their senior years, should certainly consider supplementing with the hormone progesterone, the only proven bone rejuvenator. Taken with estrogen, progesterone and a progressive weight resistance exercise schedule can quench any woman's thirst for the Fountain of Youth, especially if she takes a potent multi-vitamin and mineral capsule and sufficient antioxidants. Leg presses will strengthen the quadriceps of the thighs, plus tone the gluteus maximus muscles (your butt). Low-resistance, high repetitions will disperse hated cellulite and sculpt lean curves, while heavy-weight and low reps will promote strength and size. You are the sculptor. Weights are your chiseling tools. Space between the feet may be varied on the leg press machine, with close stance applying more stress to the vastus externus and rectus femoris and a wide stance stressing the vastus internus and sartorius for a curvaceous the thigh, (Fig. 159a). As always, a 10-1-5 cadence is most efficacious for 3 sets after a light warm-up of 25 reps. Increase the weight and drop the second set to 8 repetitions. Add more poundage for the final set of 6 reps. Barbi pushes 100 pounds for 15 repetitions. Enormous poundages are your achievable goal. I have moved from 360 a year ago to 6 reps of 630 pounds today. I watched a powerful young trainer named Ron at the BodyMasters Gym in Sandy, Utah push 1000 lbs.! Have another sip of water when you finish your set.

One-legged Extensions. For a great finish and instant final pump, try leg extensions with one leg, alternating legs with no rest between sets. Perform just 3 sets of 10 reps, one with the toes pointed forward, one with the toes pointed inward, and the final set with the toes pointed outward, all with the 10-1-5 cadence (10seconds to raise the bar, one second for holding the contraction, while you squeeze the quads, and 5 seconds to descend with negative concentration). Drink.

Squats. No exercise will build the thighs as rapidly as traditional squats, if your back can handle them. I do not recommend this exercise to seniors who are new to weight-resistance exercise. Incorrect posture can place excess stress upon the lumbar region of the vertebrae. You might also look for a gym that offers a Smith type machine which permits forward placement of the feet for greater thigh concentration.

For complete quad thigh development, use a wide stance, as opposed to a more narrow stance for rectus femoris concentration. You might want to mix up the stance for muscle confusion and resultant hyper development. Muscles become accustomed to repetitious routines, reacting with less intense response; they welcome the variety of challenges.

Allow the bar of the weight to rest on your trapezius, if it is well-developed, or use a center bar cushion. As before, begin with 25 reps and a light weight. Keep your chest inflated and high during the movement, with you back arched (never rounded). Look straight ahead throughout the movement. Descend no farther than when your thighs are parallel to the floor, (Fig. 161a). Take 10 seconds to rise during the 3 sets that follow your warm-up set of 25. Hold the contraction just before lockout for 1 second, then take 5 seconds to lower and repeat. Remember to increase the weight with each set to permit no more reps than 10 for the first set, 8 for the second, and 6 for the last. This routine, after 25 light reps, should be sufficient to stimulate anyone's thigh development, especially when it follows the first four leg exercises. Weaker readers and those whose gym time is limited should perform leg presses or squats rather than include both in the same workout. Overtraining can be catabolic. Marathon workouts which incorporate too many exercises invite free radical bombardment. We advise you to begin with the basic few I have described, but researching several physical culture magazines that are currently available, you will realize that there are many variations of the exercises I have outlined; do learn about them, as periodic change will prevent boredom and is less likely to cause perfunctory low-intensity response from the stressed muscles that are challenged.

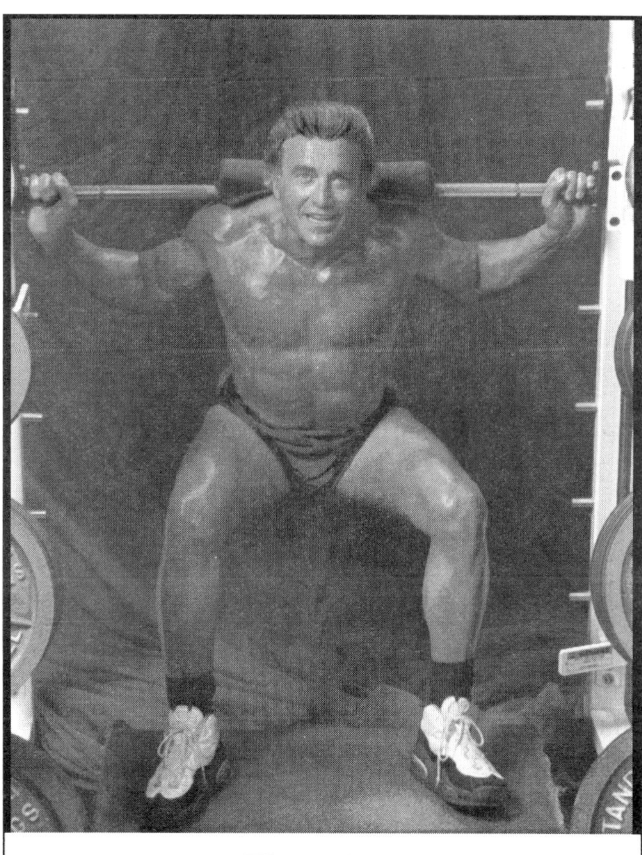

Figure 161a

Detrimental stress can be avoided by not descending too low in the Squat. The Smith machine obviates balance difficulties.

Mike Mentzer, a highly respected ex-bodybuilding champion, today recognized as a foremost theoretician of the industry, advocates a warm-up followed by no more than one set of each exercise with maximum intensity. With several different exercises designed to stress one particular muscle, such a routine is efficacious, but the key words are high intensity. Few novices will push themselves beyond the pain barrier. When I am not around, my wife reads a magazine while she does her leg extensions. High intensity demands total focus with resistance that is high enough to permit no more than the number of reps prescribed. If the set calls for 10 reps and you feel you can perform a few more, you need to increase the poundage. The last rep should always be extremely difficult.

Focus upon the working muscle can actually reward you with faster development, as focused mental concentration will isolate the contemplated muscle, forcing it to work harder. Professional bodybuilders can get away with performing fewer sets, because the steroids they inject are extremely anabolic, permitting them to use very heavy weights, and to push them beyond the pain barrier that keeps non-professionals from working out at the same intensity. Nubain, Stadol and Buprenex are the non-narcotic analgesics favored by the pros for relieving residual pain, as they mimic the effects of morphine. Buprenex has the longest duration of the three morphine analogues and also functions as a diuretic. These drugs must be prescribed, of course, and are subject to state restrictions. Few of our readers will compete in professional contests, so these drugs are contraindicated. A better choice pain reliever is a sulfur product like MSM, available over-the-counter. You can attain a rock-hard symmetrical body, drug-free, by considering our diet recommendations, scheduling potent vitamin and mineral supplementation, guarding against free radicals with the protective force of antioxidants, and submitting to hormone replacement therapy, but only if the physical program you follow includes sufficient weight resistance to induce failure beyond the prescribed number of reps. That program requires commitment and focus. Read the magazine while you "slow long distance" on the treadmill; ditch it when you train with weights. I sure hope my wife reads this.

CARDIO AND ABS DAY

Muscle is not enough to ensure your healthy journey toward maximum life span. The primary fuel is found in your cardiovascular system. When arteries clog with plaque, blood flow is constricted. The heart must be fed, and blood cannot pass through an occluded artery. What is remarkable is that the diameter of your artery is not fixed, as its girth is largely determined by the activity of the blood that flows through. Active blood flow, subject to change of pace from normal to fast to very fast and back to normal, will cause artery diameter expansion. Nature designed it that way. The wider the opening, the less likely that accumulated plaque will block the blood flow. Athletes whose lives are involved in the high-intensity interval training schedule described earlier have arteries of exceptionally large diameter, as is the diameter of their veins, which are more visible. Frank's vein diameter markedly increased during the 18 months of this book's creation. Although high saturated fat ingestion could eventually contribute to plaque lining their arterial walls, the blood of athletes would still flow normally because of the larger diameter of their arteries. All aerobic forms of exercise thus benefit the heart. The work performed in aerobic activity, therefore, is referred to as <u>cardio</u>.

Long-lasting constant activity is especially aerobic if interfered with by high intensity efforts of brief periods. Whether your chosen exercise for arterial expansion is walking, running, or spinning the wheels of a bicycle is inconsequential. I prefer the treadmill, if the weather outside is inclement; it also gives me a chance to catch up with my reading. Since a long slow cadence is most efficacious for burning fat, I pick a book or magazine that will hold my interest for 45 minutes to an hour and set the pace at 3. This setting is sufficient to raise my heart rate to 122 beats per minute, 80% of my maximum heart rate of 153 BPM (220 minus my age of 67). During that time, and always after the 16th minute, I slip into a sprint for 30 seconds that raises my BPM to near maximum. I interrupt the long slow pace 3 or 4 times with a 30-second sprint. This routine, presently once a week only, has burned a lot of fat and, hopefully, has kept my arteries from clogging, since my youthful years included a lot of butter, bread, and refined sugar. If I overdue the pasta, ice cream, or pancakes on a weekend, I include one or two more aerobic exercise periods during the week; this seems to protect my cardiovascular system from the weekend insult.

Defined abdominals seem to be the fashion rage these days. Male models are hired for their unkempt hair, pouty lips and visibly defined abdominals. Undisciplined dietary habits and neglect of aerobic activity really packed the fat onto my abdominal area, and too many beers kept my belt buckle hidden. Previously presented Figure 1 shows the result of my recalcitrance in April of 1998, the month I began to take HGH, stepped up my aerobic work, took a more scientific approach to my muscular development, and switched back to a high-protein, low-carbohydrate and fat diet. To cut down the stomach mass, I eliminated breakfast and substituted a high-protein breakfast drink which included all the major vitamins and minerals plus creatine and glutamine. Preferring the chocolate taste, I mix the drink with cold water and add a cup of hot coffee, chasing down about 15 morning vitamins, minerals and antioxidants with it. Three tabs of oat bran give me all the fiber I need, and the quick preparation gives me a half-hour extra sleep. To keep my protein ingestion high, I have another one of these drinks later in the day with hot water and glutamine, instead of coffee. I cannot handle many carbs, so I try to keep those that I do ingest of the complex variety, except for after a workout, when my glycogen has been depleted. At that time, a bottle of grapefruit juice washes down more dextrose-spiked creatine. The anabolic diet of Dan Duchaine, called Body Opus, seems to work well for me, restricting high carbs to weekends only, with a maximum of 50 grams per weekday. I am classified as blood type O, the type of Ice Age prehistoric man, and feel most comfortable eating animal, fish and fowl. We are all, of course, different, which is why we offer no prescription, just personal testimony. Previously presented Figure 2 is my testimony of six months of Spartan behavior. My strength is greater at 67 than it ever has been Yours can be, too. It is achievable.

We all have a six pack of abdominal muscles behind our flab. Lose the flab and you will find your abs. You truly do not have to work your abdominals very hard; they are there and they are beautifully shaped. You have just buried them with fat and may have stuffed yourself so much at the breakfast, lunch, and dinner tables that your stomach has distended. A low-carbohydrate, high-protein diet, fueled partly with essential fatty acids like flaxseed oil, olive oil, and EPA (fish oil), will certainly melt your fat, as your own fat will be burned for energy when you give up being a sugar-burning engine. A deliberate reduction of food volume, elimination of dairy, beer, and all starch products, and dismissal of all soda pop, will certainly shrink your stomach, sculpting even less volume. It took you years to pile on that fat; you could get rid of it in six months. My abs are still not as defined as I would like them to be, but at least I can finally see them. Can you see yours?

The abdominals are twin vertical muscles supported by a few strap-like girdles. The abs extend from the chest to the pubic area and are the major power that moves your torso toward your thighs and vice versa. While they do not require additional exercise beyond their involvement in many other exercises, some isolated tension will cause hypertrophy, if the stress is periodic and the muscles have sufficient rest and recuperation. This tension can be administered by movement of the torso toward the thighs or by movement of the thighs toward the torso. The former movement is referred to as a "sit-up," the latter as a "leg raise." These are the two principal movements, and there are many variations.

One precaution is to never extend the abdominals beyond their vertical alignment. Years ago, before bodybuilding became a sophisticated science, sit-ups were performed on "Roman Chairs," which hyper-extended the abdominals, causing many strongmen to have barrel-like guts, even though their abdominals were well developed. Today, we know that tension applied in contracted posture is all that is necessary for muscular development and can be performed even while you are driving a car for a long distance. The tension will take the boredom out of the trip, and you will arrive at your destination with an abdominal six pack that is far more socially acceptable than the six pack of beer you gave up.

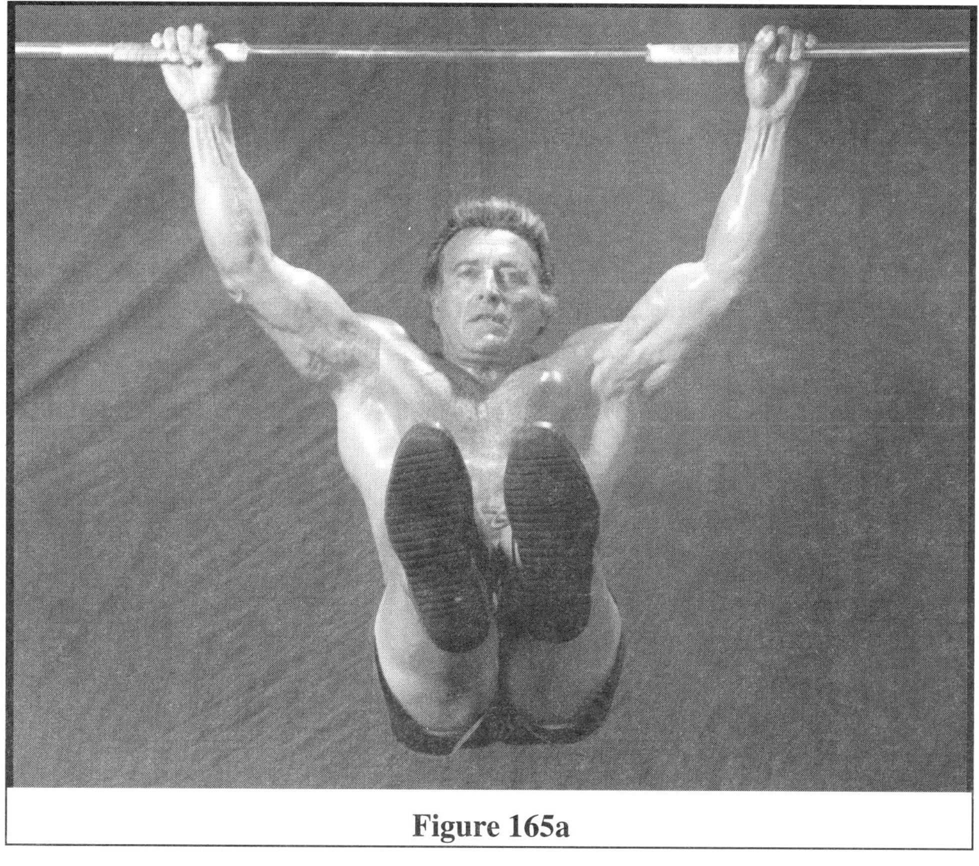

Figure 165a

Hanging Leg Raises. Some health clubs offer loop straps that support the bodybuilder from the elbows; this is an advanced movement for strong mid-sections only. You might want to try them with bent legs first.

Similar tension can be effected by raising the thighs toward the chest, on the floor or on an inclined bench. Slow and steady is still the most effective cadence: 10 seconds to rise, one second to tense the abdominal wall, and 5 seconds to return to the starting position. The same cadence works for sit-ups, too Advanced bodybuilders might try leg raises while hanging from a bar, probably the best of all abdominal exercises, as the contraction follows full extension, with gravity assisting the latter (Fig. 165a). Elbow supports are provided by some gyms for those who are grip challenged.

Sets can vary in accordance with experience, your commitment, and your strength. Just remember, it is the amount of time that you spend under tension that rips and rebuilds muscle. The abdominals are no exception. Frequency also varies according to your needs. If you have a real problem (meaning if you cannot see any semblance of the abdominal wall because of fat coverage), you could work your abdominals every day; they can take a lot of punishment.

BACK AND SHOULDERS

My favorite day. I have always coveted the V-shape of body building champions like Steve Reeves. My gymnastics experience 50 years ago is probably responsible for the foundation of this silhouette. The rings and horizontal bars were relentless in stretching the width of my upper back, every time I hung from them, but I have also been very strong with pull-down movements, much stronger than with push-up movements, when it came to training and weight resistance. From an aesthetic point of view, it occurred to me, standing at only five-foot-eight, that short men can look taller if they widened their upper back more than the lower part, the latter choice creating a short, stocky shape. The downside is that I have to order all my sports jackets and suits from Shepler's, a Western clothes store, as cosmopolitan stores cater to the square or pear-shaped male physique. It is amusing to view the difference of silhouette that can be found in city environments vs. country towns. In cosmopolitan cities today, there appear to be more V-shaped women than men. The natural design is gender specific, suggesting that form follows function. Wider pelvic bones on most women were intended for less painful childbirth. The wider shoulder girdle of most male skeletons was designed to support larger muscle for foraging, building and defending the family home. In deference to the unisex platform of the currently powerful Women's Liberation Movement, I will not extemporize that issue. Suffice it to say that even if genetic inheritance, interbreeding of different ethnic groups, and accidents of nature have made of your bone structure an aberration of natural design, you can still sculpt your silhouette with muscle development and attain any shape you desire. Conversely, lack of exercise, poor nutrition and a lethargic life style will also affect your silhouette, producing a shape that is substantially less than desirable. You are truly the sculptor of your Self. Do not blame your Creator for the shape of your body!

The V-shape necessitates development of the lateral deltoid, the latissimus dorsi, and the upper back rhomboids. As for all muscular development, the amount of time under tension that is sufficient to stress and tear the fibers of these muscles, plus the amount of time allowed for healing and recruitment of new fibers (to protect against future stress), will determine progressive development. Stress that follows a warm-up, to prepare the muscle for the trauma that will follow will be sufficient, if the exerciser follows a cadence of 10 seconds to contract, one second to hold, and 5 seconds to return to the starting position, with the provision that the weight of the challenge be increased with each set, to bring the exerciser to failure beyond the prescribed number of repetitions. Once again, contraction exercises, followed by extension exercises, will protect against muscle "binding." The first contraction exercise is the "Lat Pull-down."

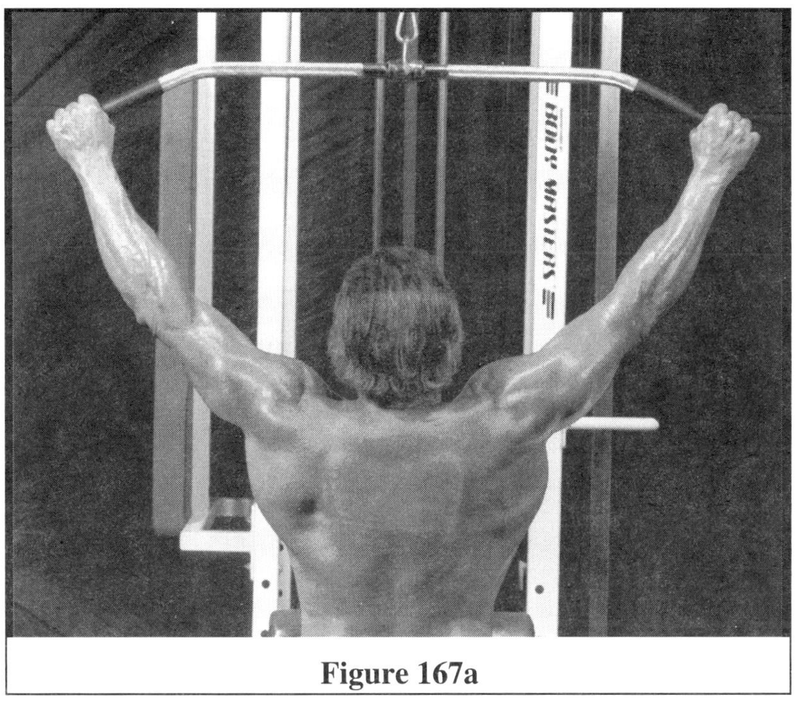

Figure 167a

A wide-grip Lat Pull-down.

Lat Pull-downs. Developing the same muscles as are stressed from "chin-ups", lat pull-downs permit the use of a resistance machine which can challenge you with less than your body weight. When you get to the stage where you can use as much weight as your body weight, you might want to switch to chin-ups, for variation. The early lat machines often required kneeling. Most contemporary machines offer a short bench for sitting. Both approaches help to isolate the back muscles without leg involvement. The biceps, of course, assist.

As usual, the warm-up should be comprised of 25 repetitions, with the set pin adjusted for light poundage (a weight that will permit no more than 25 reps). Grasp the bar with as wide a grip as you can manage. Sit and simply stretch for a minute, thrusting your chest forward (Fig. 167a). Feel your scapula bones twist and stretch the wide lateral muscles of the back called the latissimus dorsi. If there is a mirror in front of you, you will see the scapula protrusion just below and behind your armpit. Pull the bar down until it touches your pectoral

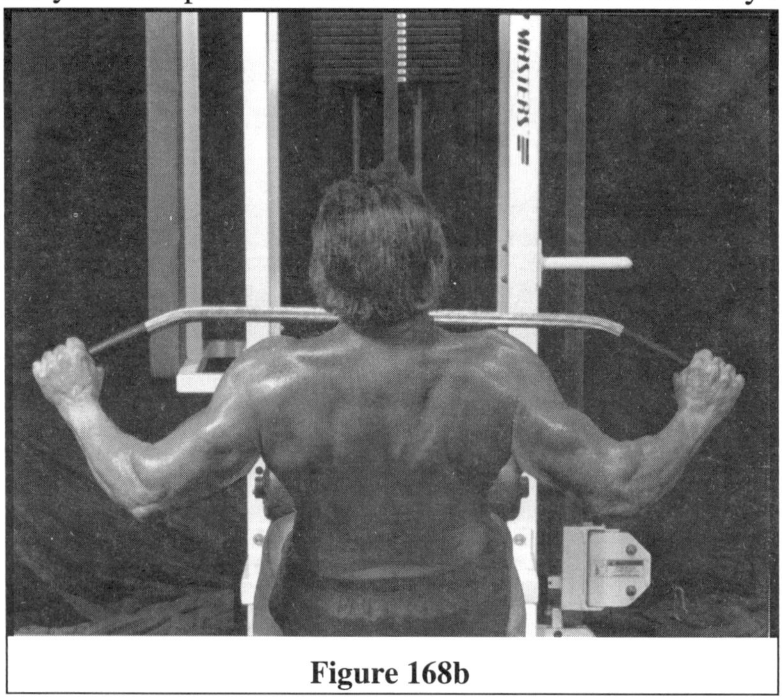

Figure 168b

Pulling the bar to your chest is preferable to pulling it to the back of your neck, if you are concerned with posture and protection of your rotator cuff.

muscles just above your nipples (Fig. 168b). Allow the bar to slowly return and continue for 25 reps. Rest for no longer than 3 minutes. Immediately proceed to the extension exercise called the "Shoulder Press."

Shoulder Presses. Years ago, only free weights were used for this vital V-shape-producing exercise. Contemporary machines take pressure off the sacrum and vertebrae, concentrating the effort in the muscles of the shoulder, called the deltoids, and the triceps of the arms. These machines have a long back support. If you are not exercising in a health club, you can use a light barbell while sitting in a chair that has a back rest. Use a weight that will permit 25 reps.

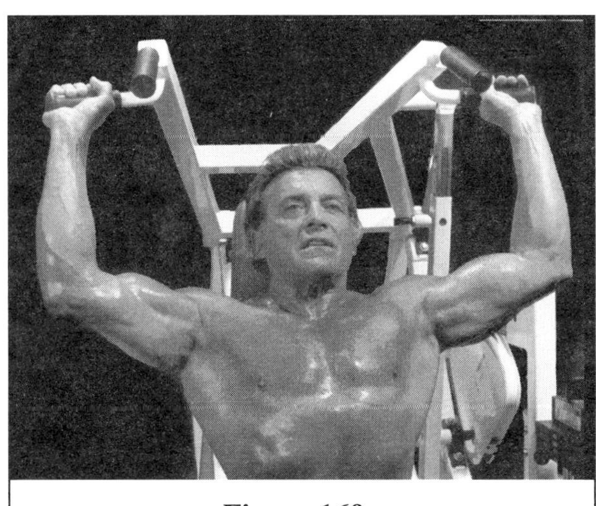

Figure 169a

Shoulder Presses while seated at a machine omit the lumbar stress that is invited when this exercise is performed standing with a barbell. Stop pressing just short of apogee on full contraction to place less stress on the elbow joint.

Grasp the handles of the shoulder press machine, or your barbell, at shoulder level with the palms of your hands facing forward. Keep the back of your hands in a straight line with your forearms (do not bend the wrists) as you press the weight slightly upward. Stop and hesitate just short of apogee (Fig. 169a) and return to the start position. Perform 25 reps of this perfect antagonist to the lat pull-downs. Rest for a few minutes. Drink.

Begin your power set of lat pull-downs next, using a weight that will permit no more than 10 reps. Failure should greet the 11th rep, or the weight shall have been insufficient. If you are new to training with weight resistance, you will need to try a test set or two to determine your personal strength level, for this and all the exercises scheduled. Perform all sets with the 10-1-5 cadence (10 seconds to press, one second to hold just below apogee, when you should squeeze the deltoid muscles, and 5 seconds to return to start position). After 10 reps, immediately proceed to the shoulder press machine or barbell for your first power set of presses.

Perform the shoulder press as before, but for only 10 repetitions with a 10-1-5 cadence Remember, if the 10th rep is easy, add more weight. You much reach failure after the 10th rep. Rest 3 minutes. Drink.

Back to the lat pull-down machine. Add more weight to greet failure at the 9th repetition. Continue the 10-1-5 cadence. Proceed to the shoulder press machine, or barbell, with no rest. Add weight to permit no more than 8 reps. Perform the 8 reps of the shoulder press with the 10-1-5 cadence. Rest 3 minutes. Drink.

The last set of lat pull-downs should be performed with a poundage heavy enough to greet failure at the 7th repetition, with the same 10-1-5 cadence. Then, proceed, without rest, to the shoulder press machine or barbell. Add weight to it to perform no more than 6 reps.

Taking 10 seconds to extend, one to tense, and 5 to return to start, you will feel an amazing pump in your deltoids. It is precisely this amount of time under tension that sufficiently stresses the muscle to tear it. During the recuperative days that follow, nature will repair the lean tissue and enlist the growth of previously dormant fiber to defend against future challenges.

Older participants may want to end their upper back and shoulder exercises here, especially if you have been away from exercise for a long time. Others should include two more variations that will strengthen the shoulder girdle and upper back.

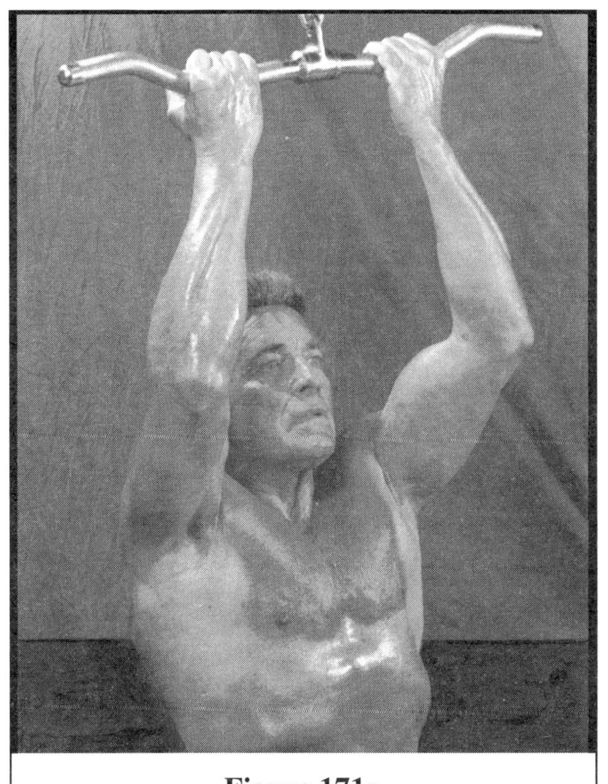

Figure 171a

Try to concentrate on the back muscles when you pull the bar down to employ their power more than the biceps of the arms. Focus can direct the effort in the Close Grip Pull-down.

Close Grip Pull-downs. Affecting central strands of the latissimus dorsi, and, of course, the biceps, is the underhanded close grip lat pull-down. Grasp the bar with your knuckles forward, allowing only 12 inches between your hands (Fig. 171a). No warm-up is necessary if you are including this and the following exercise after the first two prescribed exercises. Slowly pull the bar to your chest (take 10 seconds). Hold and tense the back muscles for a full count. Take 5 seconds to return to full arm extension. Enjoy the stretch. A variation would be to employ the same movement with one hand. Be sure to use a weight that allows no more than 10 reps. That completed, move immediately to the dumbbell rack. Select two dumbbells that will permit no more than 10 reps with each arm.

One-Arm Dumbbell Presses. These may be performed alternately (left arm, right arm, left arm, etc.) or, if you prefer, do 10 reps with the left arm, followed by 10 reps with the right arm. As we mentioned, one-arm exercises are more beneficial, as they force concentration upon one muscle at a time. More focus equals more stress, which, in turn, equals more development. Hold the dumbbell at your shoulder, with the palm of the supporting hand facing you. Slowly press the weight upward, twisting your hand as you press, to end with the palm facing forward (see Fig. 151b). The weight must be sufficient to greet failure at the 11th rep; if it is not, increase the weight. Perform 10 reps with each arm, using the 10-1-5 cadence. Then, rest a few minutes. Drink.

Follow and end your workout with two more sets of each exercise: The first set to failure after 8 reps, with a 10-1-5 cadence; rest again and finish with a set of 6 reps of each exercise, using the same slow cadence. By following every contraction exercise with an antagonistic movement, you will maintain flexibility as you develop strength.

Your first torso day is complete. Tomorrow, you will concentrate on the muscles of the chest, the posterior deltoid, and the lower latissimus dorsi.

CHEST DAY

Although the primary concentration will be on chest development, antagonistic exercises should be included to promote flexibility; these will develop the posterior portion of the deltoid and the lower strands of the latissimus dorsi. The triceps and biceps will also assist. The large muscle of the chest is called the pectoral; its fibers grow from the central sternum bone, to which your ribs are attached, and the clavicle and attach to the humerus (upper arm bone), under the deltoid.

Pectoral Flies. To stretch and contract the massive muscles of the chest, there is no more concentrated effort than that effected by what bodybuilders call flies. Flies can be performed with dumbbells on a flat bench or on a machine

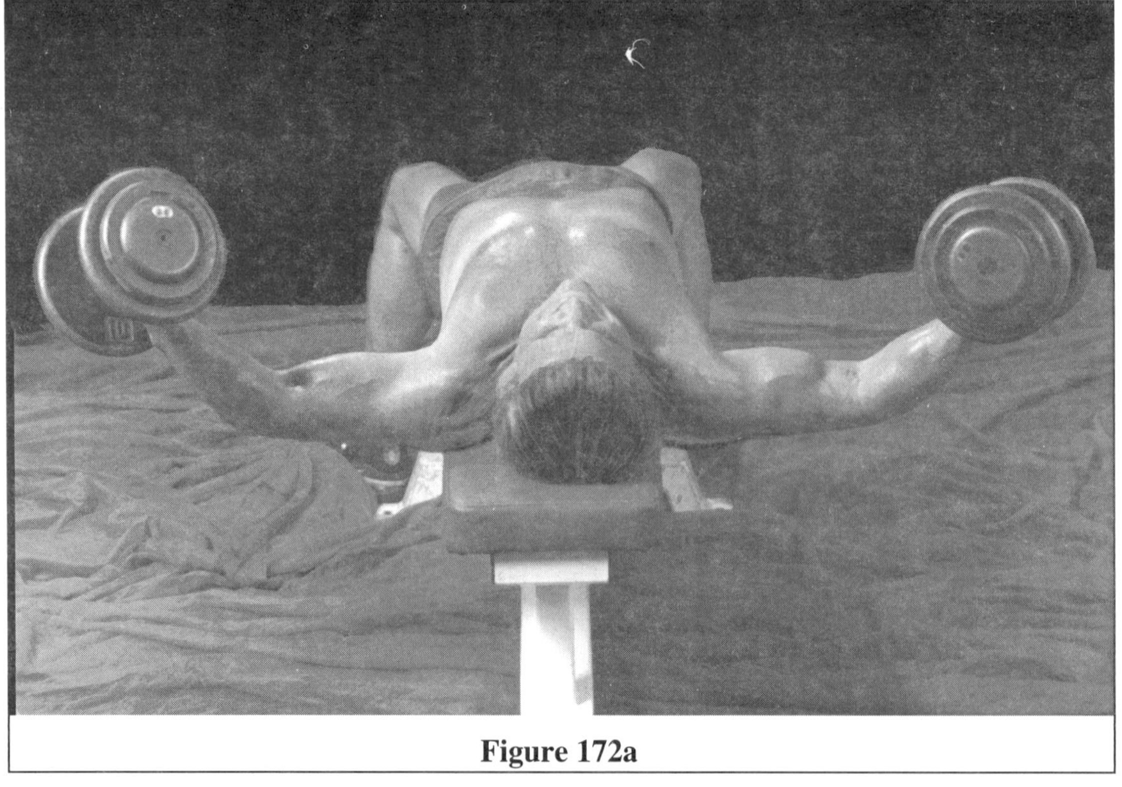

Figure 172a

A slight bend is recommended at full extension when performing Flies to avoid elbow joint stress.

called the "Pec Deck." Either movement employs full expansion and good contraction.

A. **Bench Variation**. Lie flat on a long bench with your feet flat on the ground and the dumbbells above your chest, held at full arms' length. The palms of the hands should face each other (Fig. 172a and Fig. 173b). Inhale deeply as you lower the weights toward the floor to a point just below your chest. Note the slight bend of the arms at the elbows. As always, the first set should be a warm-up of 25 reps with a light weight. Slow and steady. Take your time. Your goal is to draw blood to the chest area and volumize the cells of the pectoral muscles, in preparation for the power sets that will soon follow.

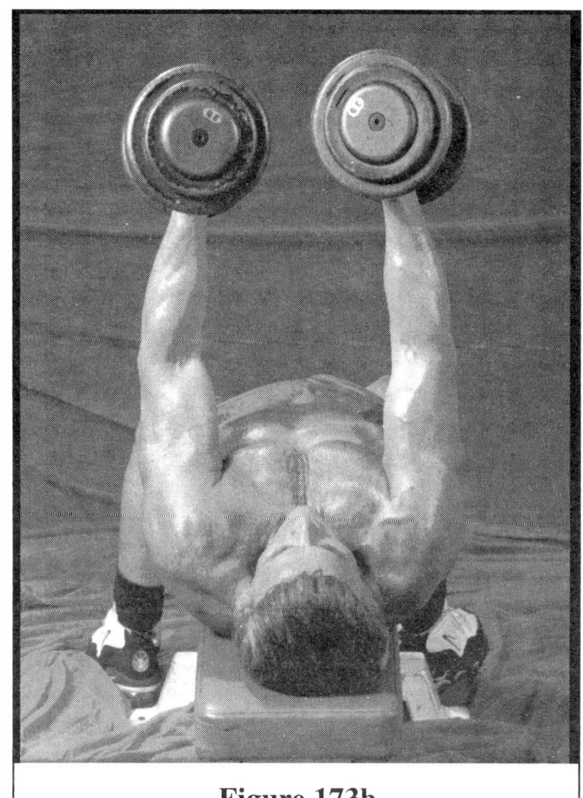

Figure 173b

The clang of kissing dumbbells is a familiar sound in the chest-developing area of most gyms, as bodybuilders face their palms to each other at complete contraction.

A. **Pec Deck Variation**. Some Pec Deck machines are set at a point which will maximize stretch of your pectorals; others offer adjustments for different arm lengths. Begin by pressing forward the pads with your forearms. Slowly advance the foam-padded handles, until your hands almost touch each other. Some Pec Deck machines allow full arm extension. Instead of forearm pads, they offer handles, which are pulled together in an arc. Hold for a contracting second and return slowly to start position. Use a weight resistance that will permit 25 reps (Fig. 174a). Focus upon your pectorals to place more stress upon them than on your biceps.

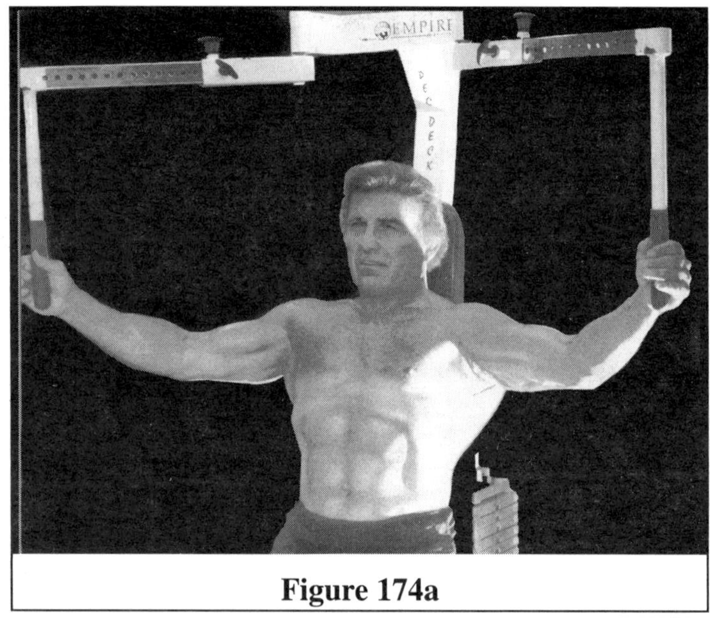

Figure 174a

Try to find a gym with a Pec Deck, like this one at the Sugarbush Sports Center, which permits almost full arm extension.

When you have completed your warm-up set of flies, either on the bench or the Pec Deck, immediately proceed to the posterior deltoid machine. If your health club does not have one, you can perform "butterflies" with dumbbells on a 45-degree inclined bench.

Posterior Deltoid Butterflies. The motion reverses that of flies to stimulate stress of the posterior deltoid, an important muscle that is underdeveloped in most people. The function of the posterior deltoid is to pull an opposing force backward with the deltoid as the fulcrum, an exactly opposite motion to pectoral flies. Some Pec Deck machines provide for either movement.

A. **Butterfly Machine Variation**. Sit facing the bench, as you reach forward to grasp the handles. Set the weight resistance to a poundage that will permit 25 reps. This is a warm-up exercise, so you need not pull to failure, but the resistance should be heavy enough to not permit many more than 25. With your deltoids as the fulcrum, pull the handles backward with only a slight bend at the elbows. The movement is similar to the swimmer's butterfly stroke. After 25 reps, rest a few minutes before moving back to your first power set of flies.

A. **Inclined Bench Butterflies**. Use this method if your health club does not include a posterior deltoid butterfly machine. Grasping two light dumbbells to permit 25 reps, lie face-down on a 45-degree inclined bench. The weakness of your dormant posterior deltoids might surprise you. Powerful bodybuilders have been surprised to find a mere 15-pound dumbbell to be sufficient. If 3 pounds defeats you before 25 reps, try a can of chicken soup in each hand. Slowly pull the weight up until your hands are almost parallel to the floor (Fig. 175a). Hold for a second and return. When 25 reps have been completely, rest a few minutes before moving on to your first power set of flies.

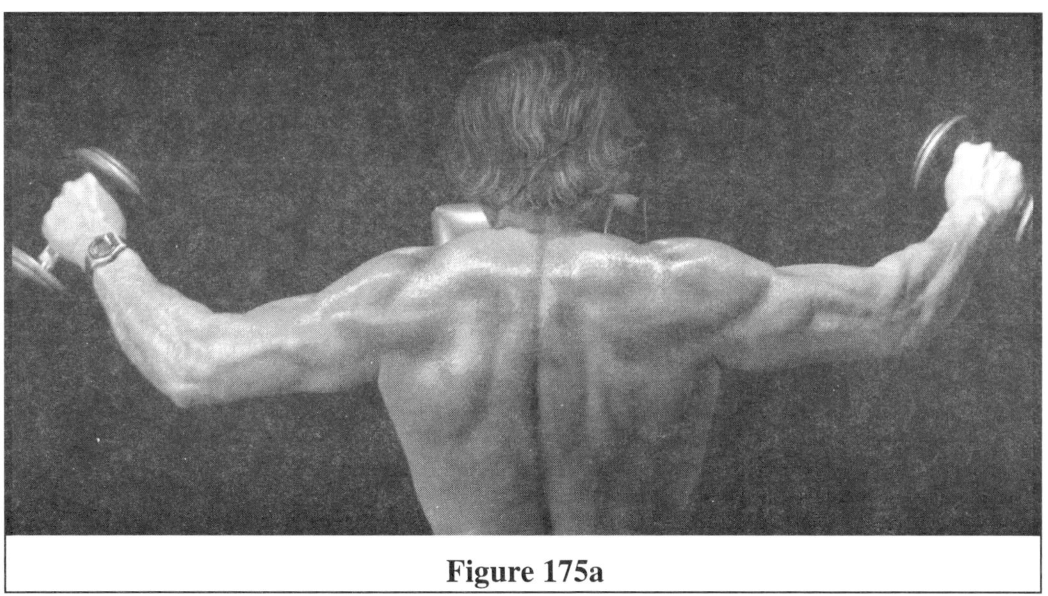

Figure 175a

Lacking a machine, this bench variation of the Butterfly exercise will quickly develop the posterior deltoid. Shown is the important stage of contraction. Hold it for a count, before taking 5 seconds to lower to start position.

The sequence for your power sets will be as follows: 10 flies, performed at a 10-1-5-cadence, immediately followed by 10 butterflies at the same cadence. In both cases, the weight must be sufficient to permit no more than 10 reps. Both sets completed, rest three minutes, then move on to your second set of power repetitions, greeting failure at the 9th rep, then do eight slow flies, followed by eight slow butterflies with no rest in between. Try for a 10-1-5 cadence, allowing your strength to determine the poundage. Do not pamper yourself. The 9th rep should be impossible; if it is not, increase the weight. When both sets are completed, have a drink of water, rest, and move on to your last power sets of flies and butterflies.

These last power sets should follow with still more weight, enough to cause failure after 6 repetitions. Using the same 10-1-5 cadence, perform 6 reps of flies and then move immediately to 6 reps of butterflies. Rest three minutes. Drink.

Bench Press. Working the pectoral mass mostly, this exercise will also enlist an assist from the deltoids and, or course, the triceps muscles of the upper arms. A flat bench stresses the entire pectoral. If a higher chest shelf is desired (more mass close to the clavicle bone), use a 45-degree inclined bench with your head at the tall end. This angle stresses the pectoral strands that connect to the clavicle more than those of the bulk of the muscle. Conversely, reversing your position, with the head lower than the hips, would enlist more of the lower fibers of the pectoral mass. Women should try all the three variations to add bulk to the muscle directly behind the breast volume. The breast, of course, is a gland that lies above the pectoral. With little or no pectoral development, the breasts will sag lower with each humiliating year. After six months of bench pressing, girls, you could throw away your bra!

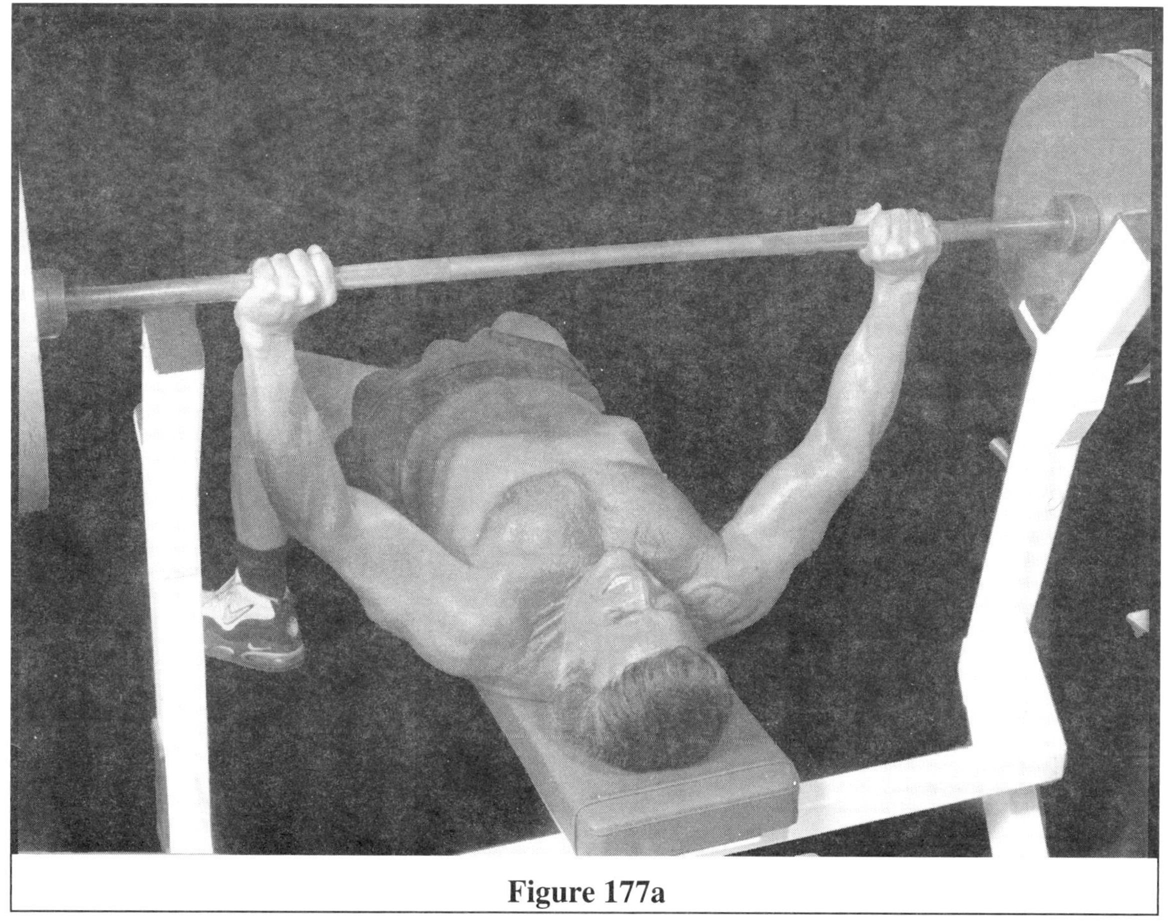

Figure 177a

Bench Press. From the holding rack, lower the bar to the bottom of the pectorals, as you inhale. Hold your breath for an instant, as you press the weight slowly upward and backward over your forehead. Hold the contraction for one second, just before full extension, then take 5 seconds to lower back to the pectorals.

The movement of the bench press is similar to the floor push-up, upside down. If you weigh over 200 pounds and you perform 25 push-ups, you should be able to press 65 pounds for 25 reps (with the provision that one-third of your body weight is in your torso). This equation would not apply to men and women who carry much more weight in their hips and legs. Women frequently do carry only one-quarter of their weight in their torso. For these women, and for men who follow suit, one-quarter of your body weight used for bench pressing warm-ups of 25 reps might better equate to 25 push-ups. Obviously, we are all different, and there are many readers who cannot perform more than 5 push-ups, due to years of torso muscle neglect. These people may require the bar alone for resistance with no added weight. Be honest with yourself, but do not pamper. Use a weight that will permit 25 reps for the warm-up set, but not many more. The movement is unusual and does stress the rotator cuff of the shoulders. Hence, the 25 rep warm-up is strongly advised, even if it requires a bar alone with no barbell plates. The macho-nerd who begins his bench presses with a heavy weight is asking for an injury that can take years to totally heal. Initially, use a barbell; lift it up and forward off its bench press rack and take 5 seconds to lower it to your lower pectorals. Slowly press the bar up and back, above your head. Just before full extension, hold for a second (Fig. 177a), and drop the bar to repeat 25 reps. Blood should rush to the region and volumize the pectorals. Breathe in as you begin to press, gradually exhaling toward extension. Now, immediately move to the lower lat pull exercise for a warm-up antagonistic set.

Lower Lat Pulls. There are three variations of this pull, all of which would reverse the bench press movement. Perform a warm-up set of 25 reps with either exercise, as they are all contracting movements, designed to balance the extension movement of the bench press.

A. **Vertical Pull-Ups**. Some health clubs offer a lat pull bench on which you may lie prone to start. Slowly pull the bar up as far as you can. Hold for a second and lower back to the starting position (Fig. 178a). Repeat for 25 reps. A variation, if no bench is available, can be jerry-rigged by placing an Olympic bar in the corner of a room, loading a plate onto the other end, straddling the bar, and grasping it just behind the plate. Be sure to bend your legs during the exercise, and do consider the use of a weightlifting belt for lower back support.

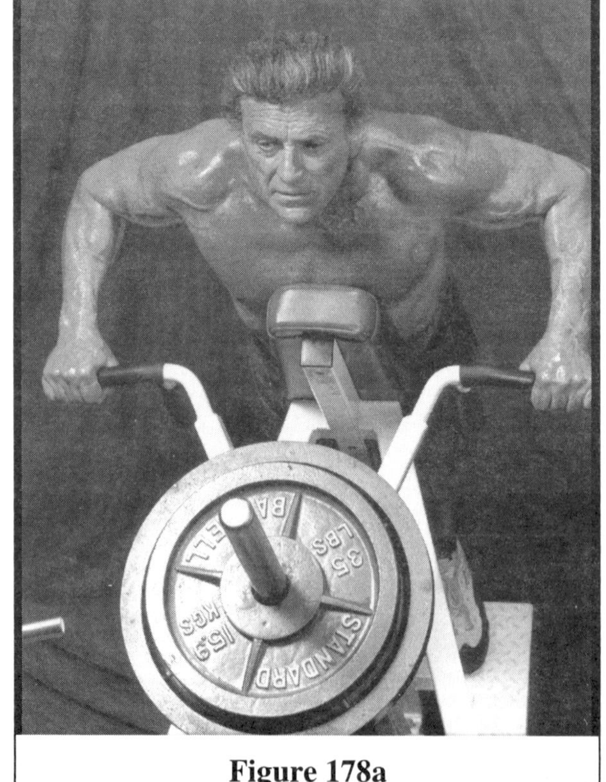

Figure 178a

A Lat Pull Bench offers an excellent variation of the Lat Pull. Keep cadence slow and hold contraction before lowering.

Use a plate that will allow 25 reps in good form.

B. **Seated Chest Pull**. A superb machine offered by sophisticated health clubs permits this excellent antagonist exercise to do bench presses with chest support. Sit with your chest against the support pad, adjusting the pad until your extended arms barely allow you to grasp the pull handles. Set the poundage pin to a weight that will permit 25 reps for your warm-up set. Pull and return slowly. Should your club not have this machine, move on to the next exercise.

C. **One-Arm Vertical Pull-Up.** For greater concentration upon the latissimus dorsi with a biceps assist, this exercise cannot be beaten and is a perfect antagonist to the muscles involved in the bench press. It is my opinion, however, that one-arm exercises are always more effective than two, if you have the time and commitment. For comfort, I like to rest my left lower leg on a flat bench and support my torso with my left fist, as I lean forward to grasp a dumbbell from the floor with my right hand (Fig. 179b). Pull the dumbbell upward with your back muscle more than your arm, until your upper arm is parallel to the floor. Use a light weight to permit 25 warm-up reps. Then, immediately switch to the left arm and repeat 25 more reps. Rest a few minutes and move on to power reps of the bench press.

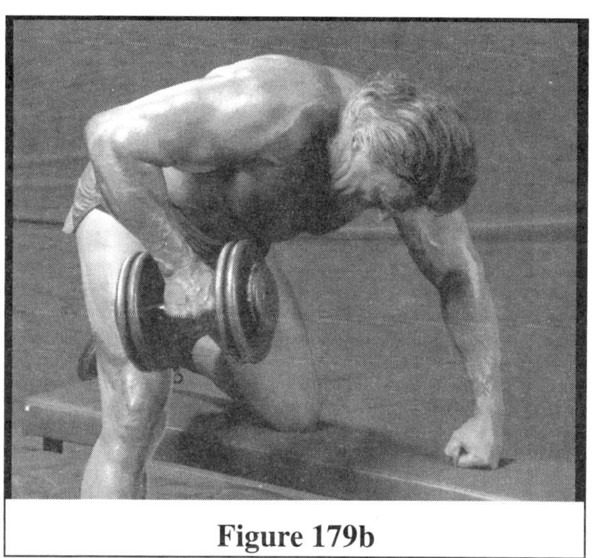

Figure 179b

One-arm Pull-Ups isolate the entire latissimus for maximum concentration. Lift weight off floor with straight arm. Focus on your latissimus when you pull the weight upward to lessen bicep movement.

After 10 power repetitions of the bench press, move immediately to one of the three variations of "pull" exercises just described. Perform a 10 repetition set with the same 10-1-5-cadence. Rest for 3 minutes. Drink, and move to your next power set of 8 reps, using the same two exercises. Finally, finish your torso day with a last set of 6 power reps. Be sure to increase the weight for each of the exercises, to work to failure after the sixth rep. Constantly focus upon the working muscle.

That will complete your 5-day workout. By the time you have reached the weekend, you will be ready for a two-day rest. You will have even more to anticipate, if you accompany the workout schedule I have outlined with the following diet.

During the 5-day workout week, I advise people I train to keep carbohydrates low (no more than 50 grams), fats at no more than 40% of total caloric intake (preferably of the unsaturated kind, like fish oil, flax oil, phosphatidyl choline, evening primrose oil and safflower), and ingest at least one gram of protein per pound of body weight. It is best to consume carbs in the morning and soon after a workout. Consider adding one or two high-protein whey drinks to your daily diet to beef up your protein ingestion. Avoid protein drinks that contain sugar. Choose a cross-filtered, ionized whey as your protein supplement. If it does not include glutamine, add it. Glutamine supplementation should not exceed 2 grams for one ingestion, but you could take that dosage 5 times daily, to stay in positive nitrogen balance. I also like to throw down a dozen desiccated liver capsules, whenever I need a protein hit for lasting energy. Creatine is optional for cell volumizing and additional strength. I loaded with 20 grams a day for the first week, then maintained with 5 grams per day. My creatine brand includes a high-glycemic additive to trigger insulin surge. Some liquid creatine products are advertised as 300% more effective, and the most recent effervescent variety claims to double that effectiveness. It tastes too sweet, but it works for me! We all respond to creatine differently. You will have to experiment to find the brand that works best for you.

Women might consider a daily hit of DHEA at no more than 25 m, to chew up the thigh cellulite. Men who are seeking rock-hard muscle mass can get these quicker with nandrolone, the highly anabolic natural hormone that can be triggered by supplementation of 19-Norandrostenediol. Try to find a brand that includes 19-Norandrostenedione, as the two seem to work synergistically via two different enzymes. The Diol version is three times as effective, so you might want to balance your dosage accordingly; 100 mg in the morning and another before retiring will create granite muscle, if you exercise to high intensity with no side effects. The prefix "nor" means without; both prohormones 19-Norandrostenediol and 19-Norandrostenedione produce nortestosterone, so you needn't worry about enlarging your prostate. For additional assurance, though, take some Saw Palmetto. For constant thermogenesis, I respond very well to the ECA cocktail (ephedrine, caffeine and aspirin) twice a day, but prefer the natural forms of these stimulants (Ma Huang, Guarana, and Willow Bark), as delivered in products like Xenadrine, Diet Fuel, Hydroxycut, and Thermodrene, all available in good health stores. Ginkgo Biloba keeps my brain alert and phosphatidyl serine protects me against cortisol-inflicted catabolism from my high-stress workouts. I also employ a host of antioxidants to attack the free radicals that accompany my thirst for oxygen after aerobic activity; these include vitamin E, C, Pycnogenol and Co-Q-10 for my heart.

Yes, I am a pill freak, have been for over 25 years, and I've taken a lot of teasing for the dozen that supplement my breakfast and the dozen that boost the nutrients from my dinners. But some of those laughing non-believers are now suffering from emphysema, osteoporosis, atherosclerosis, and other debilitating diseases, which they conveniently blame on their age, and they are all considerably younger than I. Sure, I have spent a bundle on supplements, but have saved a bundle by not smoking, avoiding smoky pits of iniquity like the local bars, and by living in a pure-air rural area, where I can wear blue jeans and not have to worry about whether my three-button suit had a more expensive designer than my neighbor's. The cost of good health is surprisingly small, when you compare it to the cost of pretentious property. It is a question of values.

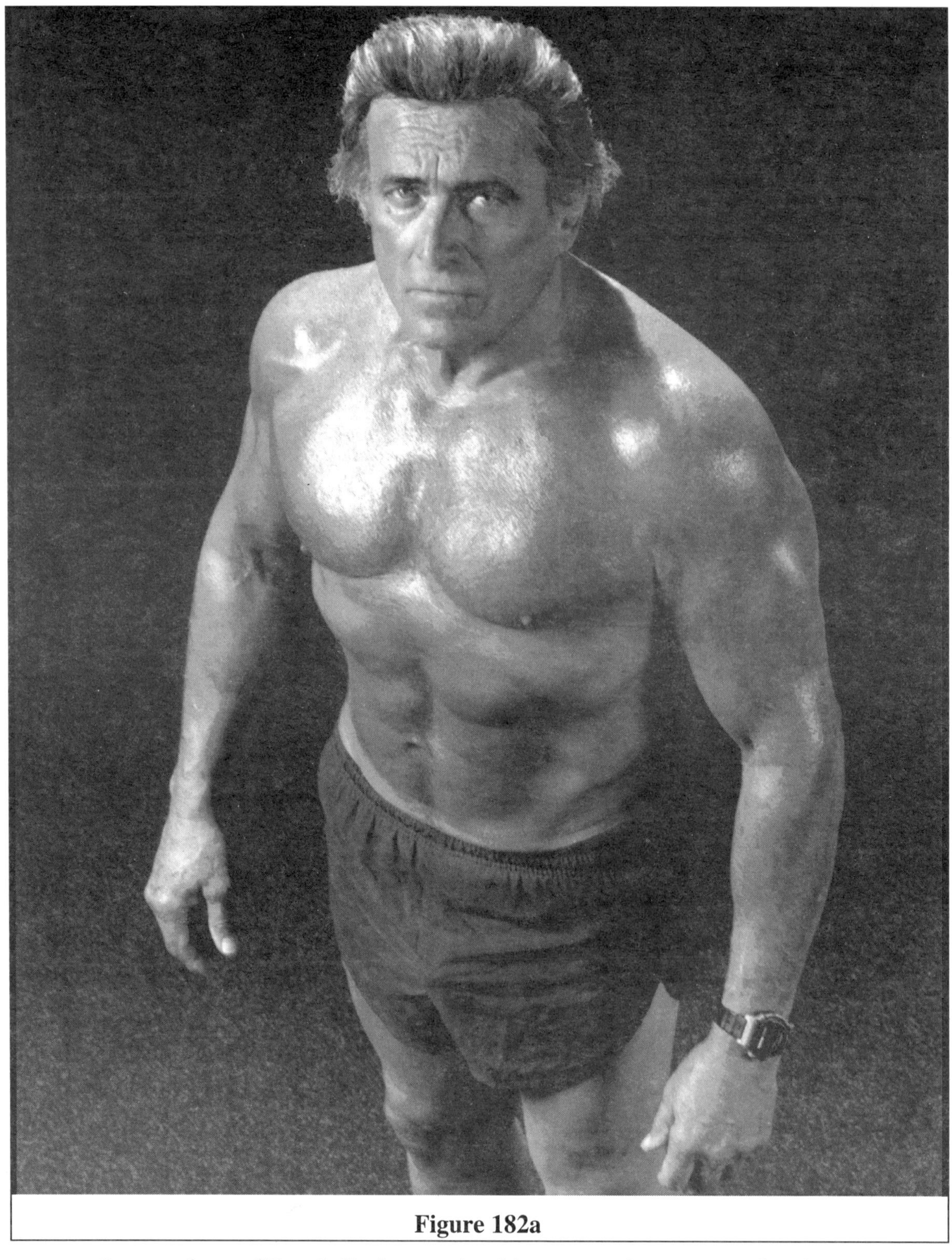

Figure 182a

Recent photo of Frank Covino venting his rage against age at a local gym.

Time for another disclaimer, since we live in a such a litigious society: This course in physical fitness is not a prescription for you, but merely an outline of the program that has worked most effectively for an author who has begun his 68th year and is stronger and more productive than he has ever been (Fig. 182a). That is worth more to me than a par 69, a national tennis trophy, or a Ferrari. Again, it is a question of values.

Chapter Four

Fighting Psychological Stress

Brain Boosters And Mental Enhancers

"Be all that you can be." I am sure we all recognize this as the United States Air Force recruitment slogan. But if we want to be all that we can be in the golden years, we must pay special attention to our brain as well as to our body.

If you have ever spent frantic moments searching for misplaced keys, gotten lost while following directions from memory, or have become lost for a word in the middle of a conversation, then you know how annoying or frightening a lapse of memory can be. For millions of older people, this is a way of life. Frank calls it "a senior moment."

To understand how we can boost our brain power and enhance our mental abilities, we must recognize that our brains are the most complex, specialized, magical organs in our bodies. The brain is the second-largest organ in our body, second only to our skin, and is also the heaviest. The brain has many varied functions, coordinating all of the body's nervous activity, processing incoming sensory impulses, as well as being the hub or reasoning, intellect, memory, emotions, and consciousness. Our brains require constant nourishment from oxygen and nutrients, and if deprived of these, within minutes brain cells begin to die, and death of the brain's host is inevitable. The brain is the organ most affected by oxidation and damaging free radical activity, these being one of aging's most significant causes.

Brain cells are called neurons, and they communicate with one another by releasing chemicals called neurotransmitters along a vast network of branch-like cells called dendrites. As one ages, there is a decline in neurotransmitters and dendrite formation of as much as 60% to 70%, thereby explaining the reason for memory lapses, difficulty in learning new things, and loss of our psychic energy.

Dr. Anderson has successfully treated hundreds of patients with complementary prescriptions such as these which follow; consider them in lieu of drug regimens prescribed by mainstream physicians.

How We Can Improve Our Brain Power

1. **Diet:** Drink 5 ounces of water for every 10 pounds of your bodyweight daily. To combat the oxidation and free radical activity, our diets should be rich in antioxidants obtained from fruit, vegetables and grains, or from antioxidant supplements. Also, a healthy diet should be composed of low saturated fat, moderate complex carbohydrates, and moderate to high protein, the level of the latter raised in accordance with activity intensity. There is no nutrient value in simple carbohydrates, especially from processed sugars and "refined" starches. Eliminate them.
2. **Consider necessary micronutrients daily in the form of vitamins, mineral and herbal supplements:**
   - Antioxidants - Vitamins A, C, E to fight damaging free radicals. Alpha lipoic acid (100 mg) and Co-Q-10 (50 mg).
   - Potent B-complex (100 to 150 mg) supplemented with 500 mg of niacin, B2, B6, B12 and folic acid.
   - Ginkgo Biloba (40 mg extract) - To increase microcirculation, thereby flushing nutrients and oxygen to the brain.
   - Proanthocyanidins (30 mg) like Pycnogenol (derived from grapeseed extract and pine bark extract) are powerful antioxidants and free radical scavengers.
   - Phosphatidyl serine (200 mg) - Supports cell membrane integrity and combats cortisol, preventing catabolism.
3. **Supplement with anti-aging hormones and prohormones, if your levels are low** (see *Chapter Two* for more detailed information):
   - Melatonin
   - Pregnenolone
   - Thyroid
   - DHEA
   - 19-Norandrostenediol and 19-Norandrostenedione (time-released),
   - Testosterone
   - Estrogen and Progesterone
   - Human Growth Hormone (based on your IGF-1 level)
4. **Exercise the brain**:
   - It is important to exercise your brain. We have learned that by challenging ourselves mentally at any age, we can build new nerve connections and strengthen neuron pathways.

- Brain workouts. Make it a point to read, play word games (Like Scrabble or crossword puzzles), and learn something new each day. Throw away your calculator.
- Challenge your brain by acquiring a new skill. Learn to dance, paint, play an instrument, take educational classes at local colleges in your community, learn karate or yoga, take up gardening. The median age of students enrolled in the Frank Covino Academy of Art is 50. Many of his students have become proficient realistic oil painters after retirement age; some are earning extra income from their newly discovered brain exercise.
- Turn off thc TV, a dangerous captivator of brain energy that can destroy your creative potential. If you must be entertained by the boob tube, limit your time to news and educational programs, and especially guide your children, who are strongly influenced under the spell of this hypnotic instrument.
- Listen to talk radio.
- Listen to classical music which has been proven to grow healthier plants, while the popular nihilistic music of the late 20th century has been proven to kill them. Wise Vermont farmers have learned that classical music results in sweeter, more plentiful milk from their cows.
- Have social interactions. Visit friends, volunteer in your community, help those less fortunate, but do not discount the benefits of meditative solitude.

5. **Exercise your body**. Physical exercise increases the amount of oxygen and nutrients available to the brain, by making the heart strong and increasing the heart rate. During exercise, we also have the release of friendly neurochemicals like endorphins and dopamine, creating a "natural high" and increased sense of well-being. Constant physical exercise taxing the heart at 75% of its maximum rate for at least 30 minutes, 3 to 4 times per week, can be a major factor in keeping our brains stimulated and youthful.
6. **Eliminate brain toxins**. These toxins are known to interfere with our natural brain chemistry, affecting memory and alertness. Included are recreational drugs like marijuana, cocaine and amphetamines, beta-blockers, used to treat high blood pressure, pain killers, daily antihistamine use, diet pills, antidepressants, tranquilizers, sleeping pills, alcohol abuse, nicotine, and high-saturated fat or high-sugar diets.

The Role and Use of Prescription Medications Known as Smart Drugs

Smart drugs have been around for a long time and have had numerous studies to support their effectiveness and safety, if natural substances like lecithin, Ginko Biloba, and phosphatidyl choline fail. The three most commonly used "smart drugs" designed to boost brain power are deprenyl, hydergine, and piracetam.; these, of course, need to be prescribed by a qualified physician.

Deprenyl, also known as Elderpreyl or Seleguline, slows down production of monoamine oxidase B, (MAO), a naturally, but sometimes overly produced, substance as we age. It has been implicated in Parkinson's disease and aging of the brain. Studies have shown that deprenyl increases the availability of the neurotransmitters dopamine, norepinephrine, and phenylalanine, playing a major role in cognitive motor and behavior functions. In studies of rats with induced Parkinson's disease, researchers serendipitously found that deprenyl improved memory, boosted cognitive function, increased sexual vigor, and increased their life span by about 40% compared to untreated rats. Today, deprenyl is also used by many neurologists and alternative physicians for Parkinson's and Alzheimer's disease, to improve the quality and productivity of patients afflicted with these conditions.

Hydergine was originally prescribed as an overall vasodilator for increasing blood flow to the brain and lowering blood pressure. Patients being treated with this medication noted marked improvement in their mood, memory, and cognition. Hydergine enhances brain activity through the following:

1. Increases blood flow, thereby increasing oxygen and nutrients supplied to the brain.
2. Raises serotonin levels in the brain.
3. Increases protein synthesis and nerve growth factor.

Piracetam is a cerebral stimulant that appears to have an effect on the cerebral cortex and related structures, without any of the side effects normally produced by other cerebral stimulants. Piracetam has a number of distinct properties:

1. Protects brain against damage from oxygen starvation (hypoxia) and enhances brain recovery from such an event.

2. Increases rate of metabolism and energy level of brain cells.
3. Enhances learning and memory in healthy volunteers as well as in memory-impaired people.
4. Protects against memory loss from physical injury and chemical poisoning.
5. Facilitates transfer of information between the two halves of the brain.

These smart drugs are, as we mentioned, only available by prescription. Consult with your doctor to learn if you are a candidate for such treatment. With an effective exercise program such as we have outlined and the diet and supplements that we have listed, you should not need any prescription drugs.

Mind/Body Interaction

A basic premise in mind/body medicine is that chronic stress and lack of balance contribute to illness. Chronic stress plays a major role in premature aging of the brain. From the "fight or flight" reaction that we have to perceived danger, there is a definite physiological response to chronic physical and emotional stress, causing the release of stress hormones like adrenaline and cortisol. These hormones quickly flood our brain and body to initiate a cascade of physiological defenses, putting us in to a hyper-alert, energized state, ready to take action. The older we are, the greater the negative impact these hormones have on our body, accelerating brain damage. I am sure we all can relate to being over-stressed due to our fast-paced life and over-commitment, experiencing forgetfulness, inability to concentrate, and difficulty with appropriate word retrieval. If stress contributes to accelerated aging, then stress reduction should promote active health and longevity. Clearly, we need to find "stress busters" to promote physical and mental relaxation and prevent premature aging of our brains. Following are some techniques or simple solutions to help alleviate stress and enhance our spirit.

1. **Exercise.** Even if it only consists of a brief walk for 10 to 20 minutes, exercise can have a major impact on decreasing stress hormones as well as bringing about the release of endorphins and dopamine to give us a natural high or calming effect. Interrupt that walk with a short sprint and you will exercise your most important muscle, your heart. Consider the regimen outlined in *Chapter Five*. You'll feel rejuvenated.
2. **Meditation**. Learn this ancient contemplative technique, and within 10 to 15 minutes, you can place your mind in a peaceful state. Consider the power

of private prayer. Explore foreign forms of contemplation. Try some Tai-Chi. Turn off your Walkman.

3. **Aromatherapy**. Reduces stress through the power of scent for relaxation and mental peace. Enjoy the healing smells that soothe your walk through a forest. Travel as far as you must to smell the ocean at least twice a year.
4. **Socialize**. Some social life is important for nurturing the human spirit, the contact which may be necessary for staying healthy and vibrant. Choose your friends wisely, though. Losers beget losers. Doomsayers beget depression. Hug an optimist.
5. **Avoid debt**. Consolidate those charges to one card and burn the others. Choose the credit card with the least amount of interest; pay it off and burn it.
6. **Live in the present moment**. Do not commiserate over regrets of the past or be fearful of the future. As Frank has written in the chapter dealing with psychological distress, disappointing events end one chapter of your life, but they also begin another.
7. **Choose to have a positive attitude**. Your cup can be half-empty, unless you choose to view it as half-full. Optimists live longer than pessimists.
8. **Take frequent breaks or mini-vacations**. Every engine needs a periodic tune-up.
9. **Let no man, woman, or child control your life**. Choose a mate who wants to share your life and be sure that you reciprocate by supporting your mate's interests. Many contemporary homes are run by the youngest family members. Be a servant to your child, and they will soon disrespect your frailty and lack of assertiveness. You cannot buy love with servitude. Respect is earned from a show of strength and accomplishment.
10. **Live in, or at least frequently visit, a healthy clean air environment**. Are you trading health for urban pretentious sophistication? This is a big country. How much of it have you seen? You do not necessarily have to live where your parents settled.
11. **Create something.** Anything. Such creation will elevate you above non-creative animals. Animals can make babies, but they cannot knit, carve, paint, or create music.
12. **Love someone**. Unconditionally. Whole-heartedly. Find something to love in everyone, beginning with yourself. Love begets life. Poet D.H. Lawrence advises us to transmit life, for when we fail to transmit it, life will fail to flow through us. Read his poem, "We Are Transmitters" (1928).

13. **Discover generosity**. Another trait that will distinguish you from animals.
14. **Forgive without resentment**. Tough call, but a sure road to inner peace. Work on it.
15. **Adopt a friendly cat or dog**. Pets have been proven to lower blood pressure and tranquilize the brain. Just do not choose a big dog if your neighbor has a small cat.
16. **Buy a canoe**. Discover a tranquil lake at sunrise or sunset, the most beautiful times of the day. Share it with someone special, or enjoy the placid contentment of solitude, in tune with the harmony of nature's quiet sounds. No church can bring you closer to God.
17. **Read this book**. And then share it with a friend, so that you may both apply its principles.

Someone more eloquent than your authors has wisely advised, "Today is the beginning of the rest of your life…"

Your Self and Its Role in Society

Brain-booster supplements can certainly keep us alert and productive in our senior years, especially when those just mentioned are complemented with a potent daily vitamin and mineral regimen, a properly balanced diet, and weight-resistance exercise. But a strong, necessary part of the equation in our quest for active longevity is psychological balance. Awareness of the Self and how it is affected by the roles it plays in society is necessary to combat the cortisol that is secreted whenever our psyche is confronted by a situation of mental stress. Debilitation from years of adversarial attacks is cumulative and can end with termination of the Self, if a lifetime of erosion leaves little to combat the final insult.

It has occurred to the author that the only way to defend against a lifetime of psychologically damaging insults is to keep the core of the Self separate from the roles we play in the social theater, loaning pieces of it to each of those assignments (in order of degree of importance), striving for excellence of performance, but cautiously never surrendering our complete Self to any one of those roles. Total commitment of the Self to any one role, often surrendered naively and with generous motive, can lead to destruction of the Self, should the role be terminated. Such annihilation has been referred to with euphemisms ranging from "nervous breakdown" to "dementia." Our goal, to remain healthy through the last day of our lives, can only be realized if we maintain a strong psyche, so this problem of social contact needs to be addressed.

Imagine your Self as the center of a vast galaxy, the fiery sun that charges each of its orbiting planets with vital energy. Allow each planet to represent one role played by you in society, placed in an orbit determined by its importance. Thus, if your principal role is that of Mother, assign that office to the planet that is in closest orbit to your Self. Assign your second most important role to the planet of the next closest orbit, perhaps Wife. Each subsequent role should then be relegated to its own orbit, in order of importance to your Self, i.e., Artist, Nurse, Corporate Executive, Teacher, Housekeeper, Activist, Member of Religious Order, and so on. Extroverts will probably list a vast universe; introverts may document a small one, but you have the rest of your life to expand it.

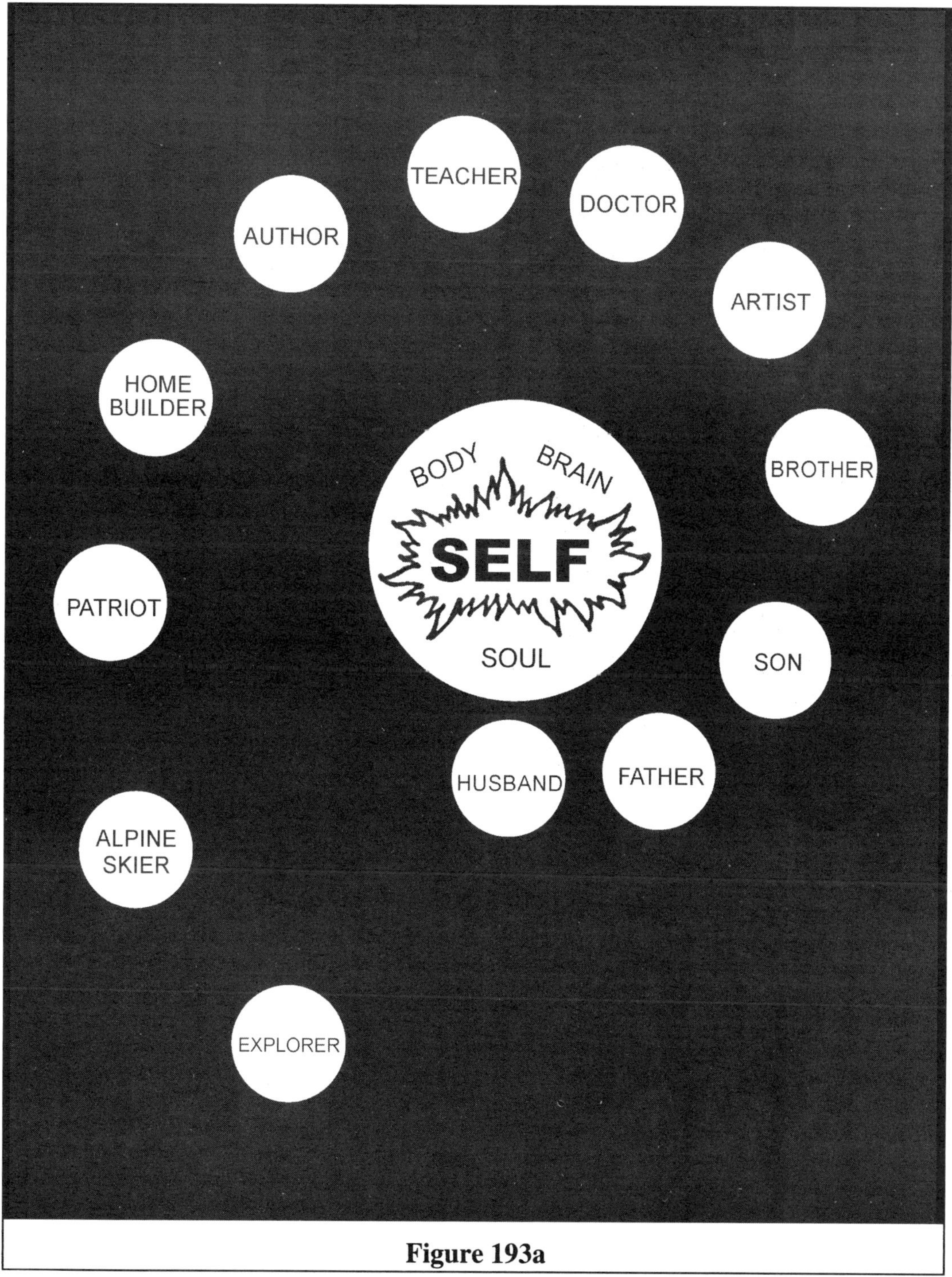

Figure 193a

While the central energy force of the Self is comprised of body, brain, and soul, we all differ in the amount of potential development in each of these categories. Sketch your own interpersonal relationship "galaxy," with each "planet" in an orbit related to your estimation of importance. Be cautious, though. Total surrender of your Self to any one of these special roles can result in Self-annihilation, if that role is terminated.

Planets are dependent upon their central energy source, their sun, for survival. The existence of that sun is not dependent upon any of its planets. The roles you play in society depend on the energy of your Self. What we need to realize is that the Self is not dependent on any one of them. What would happen to your Self if you totally surrendered it to one of your social roles and some terrible event terminated that role? Your Self would die with it, of course; if drugs or booze did not finish the job, debilitating diseases and early mortality would soon follow the resultant stress. Even the responsible roles of Mother or Father are susceptible to this hypothetical, tragic chain of events. If you were to surrender your entire Self to the role of Parent, and a traumatic event suddenly causes the death of your child, your Self would perish, too. Two lives can thus be wasted from one tragic event. You may continue to exist, but you will not be living. Honkey-Tonk bars are full of wasted selves. Some of these people lost a mate; others a child; some have lost both. My mother lost her first child. She could have ranted and raged over the injustice, drowning her sorrow in booze. Instead she prayed for strength, courage, and understanding, and was rewarded with three more healthy children. Women seem to cultivate broader universes, exploring new planets as fast as former ones explode. Many 20th century men channel all of their energies toward one role (the role that returns the most income), risking annihilation of their Self, should the role terminate.

For example, ranch women are the central energy source of vast galaxies. When the closest city is 100 miles away from the ranch, there is little choice but to be self-sufficient and devote portions of the Self to many roles. In close orbit to the Self of a Texan ranch woman is the role of Wife, closely followed by Mother, then Grandmother (although I have known some to reverse the order at menopause). These most important roles are followed by dozens of essential roles that are necessary to be the principle energy source of a ranch, with relatives, ranch hands, and animals all dependent on them. Yet they still find time for creative roles like oil painter, knitter, rug maker, quilter, pottery designer, etc. The American ranch woman, with her diversified interests and creative energies, is not unlike the Renaissance Man; it is probably more than a coincidence that both were energized by strong faith. Dr. Anderson and I feel most fortunate in having married such physically and mentally active women. Neither of us could be as productive without their support. Barbi's principal anxiety is that there is not more time to paint. She is a superb artist, so I can feel that pain. If this were the Renaissance, we might be painting every day. But painting and sculpting were highly respected arts in that era, and gifted artists were subsidized. There were also no deadlines. Yet, Leonardo is proof that the greatest artists from that period were also diversified. There are only ten paintings in the world that we know were created by da Vinci. What did he do with the rest of his time? History reveals that this incredible genius was principally an inventor (the hang glider, parachute, bicycle, submarine, clocks, contact lens, incredible weapons of war, and so on), who worked as an engineer, architect, and sculptor. If we can believe Vasari, this brilliant Italian artist was also physically fit enough to win Florentine sports contests and, as I have mentioned elsewhere, strong enough to open a horseshoe with his bare hands.

Few women would respond to her doctor's grim announcement of terminal cancer the way Texan ranch woman, Elvie, did (L.V. is short for her Christened name, Lillian Vanilla). The doctor gave her "about a year" to live. Her ranch outside of Sonora is not too far from the Mexican border. "No jump for a jumper," she would say. She had heard that Mexican doctors had been treating cancer patients with Laetrile and a potent vitamin and mineral supplement regimen with great success. Neither cure has been recognized by the AMA in our country. Her husband, Jack, had died, so after leaving a cancer-laden piece of herself on the operating table, Elvie packed her Suburban and headed for the border.

That was over 15 years ago. Today, she is one of my most loyal art students, attending workshop seminars in many different states. If Elvie had not diversified her interests, if her entire Self had been surrendered to the one role of wife, when Jack was called, she might have soon followed. She fulfilled every obligation of her marital partnership, raising two beautiful children, who have both given her grandchildren. Jack's passing was painful, of course. Together they had accumulated 11 sections of land (one section = 640 acres). I helped Elvie herd her cashmere goats not too long ago, then asked if I could keep the horse for another hour to ride to the end of the property. She smiled an okay. By nightfall, I still had not found a fence!

In addition to her ranch roles, Elvie has been a trained, licensed pilot, a dressmaker, a fantastic cook, a carpenter, and, after 14 years of study and practice, a portrait painter in the Classical tradition. Approaching the sagacious age of 80, she is an inspiration to the students of every class she attends. Elvie has learned to delegate portions of her Self to many roles, never totally surrendering the core. If any of those roles terminate, she will have plenty of her Self left for new assignment. Much as with any form of sound investment, diversification seems to be the key to survival.

Corporate workers especially should be careful. We have a friend who is an incredible survivor. Bryan has been known to give an enormous percentage of his Self to close orbiting roles like Husband, Father, and Corporate Employee. So loyal was he to the Fortune 100 Corporation which employed him, that he would take work home each night to improve his efficiency. His dedication rewarded him with a shocking dismissal, when some marketing expert convinced the company they could profit from "laying off" a large number of employees, investing in computer technology to take their place. Such brutal termination is common in the corporate world of today in the name of industrial progress. There was, at least, some severance pay which helped salve the wound, but the ungrateful act put Bryan out of work for more than a year.

Debts piled up. His blood pressure soared, and beer became a familiar companion. Tension developed between him and his wife, despite Bryan's devoted effort toward his role as Husband, working day and night to build a comfortable home for his family. Angry voices soon destroyed the peaceful union and the words "for better or worse" were soon forgotten. His wife left him, taking their two baby boys. So much for the last line of the marriage contract, "until death do us part." There are no guarantees.

Just one of those disappointments, both a painful psychological insult, would be enough to destroy many men. But Bryan is a man of faith, and, although Canon law of the religion he was born into condemns a man for divorcing and remarrying, he appealed to a higher authority (the Most High) for understanding, compassion, and the strength to extinguish his natural resentment. As a friend who has been visited by similar distress, I suggested that he reassess the worth of his Self, end this chapter of hurt and grief, turn the page, and get into the next chapter. He did.

Not to divorce, in a relationship of hopeless conflict, is to take the road toward sickness and early mortality, as the resultant stress will be compounded. With the entire Self surrendered to such a destructive union, the pain brought by stress will be constant and relentless, mutilating the Self repeatedly, until total destruction brings the peace of final breath. Some of my students are married to brutal husbands, who feel they have license to humiliate, subjugate, and ridicule with verbal and physical abuse. These women know pain, but they stay married because of religious doctrine or "for the sake of the children." No just God would ever condone such abuse. No child could ever benefit from witnessing such cruelty. No frocked man, who has never married, can possibly understand the stress of sexual anxiety, domestic strife, and conflict. No celibate socially inexperienced man should have the right to condemn divorce. The Thomas Mertons make the best priests.

I do not know any man who has given more of himself to his wife and family than Bryan. I know no man who has been as loyal and as dedicated to his employer. Both separations seriously eroded what was left of his Self, but, fortunately, there was enough left for him to follow my advice and listen to the wisdom expressed in a popular song by another Frank: "That's life...You've gotta pick yourself up, and get back in the race!" Several years later, Bryan has a better job, with a company that recognized his diligence and loyalty. He has a new wife, who is truly an angel, and joint custody of the children he bred. We are still working on the resentment.

The role of Husband has eluded our friend Pat. If honesty, loyalty, intelligence, strength, and affable nature were the first things woman looked for in their attraction to men, he would have no problem; they describe him perfectly. At the tail end of the 20th century, it appears that women's values in their attraction to men are rather shallow. Among teenage girls, good looks rank first; *cool* runs a close second (a reflection of dress, hair style, manner, and attitude that the Gods of Teendom, rock music stars, deliver on MTV). Older women, perhaps scarred from disillusioned experiences with boys of such meaningless attributes, opt for money, another false God that promises security but seldom brings happiness. Pat was blessed with none of these female-attracting qualities. His pock-marked face and prodigious nose caused a constant barrage of psychological insults throughout his youth, but Pat had strong faith.

That faith took what was left of his psychologically scarred Self and applied a huge chunk of it to his participation in a new sport. The sport did not necessarily involve competition; it invited male and female participation at any age; it was outdoors, far away from industrial pollution; it called for agility, focus, and elegant grace, but asked for no hit and conquer, and there were no scores. Pat became proficient at the sport of skiing; so well did he perform on snow that in a short time, he earned the highly respected title of Examiner for the Professional Ski Instructors of America (PSIA). A major achievement, the role orbited his Self in close proximity and became his sole universe. Each year Pat came closer to delivering what Plato would have called the Perfect Form.

Total Self-commitment had rewarded Pat with a huge planet, but there were no other planets in the galaxy.

Springtime lures many Eastern skiers from southern areas to the high country of Vermont, so it was no surprise when Pat called us at Sugarbush Valley to pop up for a visit. Headed north on Route 91, he pulled his station wagon under an overpass, dropped the tailgate, sat, and enjoyed the warm rays of the sun, while he munched a tuna sandwich. Screeching tires and the crunch of metal interrupted his meditation. Pat looked up to see a demolished car diving from the overpass and heading straight for him. He does not remember much about the hours that followed, but will never forget the horror of awakening in a Massachusetts hospital with a short stump of what used to be his leg.

We had not heard about the accident. A year passed with no word from our friend. When he arrived on crutches for a surprise visit, my heart stopped. I looked down at the stump, up at Pat's eyes, red and clouded with tears, and then away from him, as though, if I looked away the tragedy would be erased. Then, I felt anger. How, in the name of mercy, could God take away the only joy this man ever experienced in his life? I might have gone on to more blasphemous thoughts, if I had not seen the pain in Pat's face and had not heard the suicidal conversation that followed. There was, in his heart, no reason to go on. Skiing was his life. I sensed that he had come this time to say goodbye. I had to think fast.

"Pat, you were the best American skier that I've ever known. I think about your precision every time I carve a turn. You were gifted with that talent to inspire hundreds of other ski instructors. We trembled to be tested by you, but were honored to have been influenced by your guidance. You were put here for a purpose, and that mission may only now be revealing itself." As I spoke, I secretly prayed for the right words; when they came, I felt embarrassment and guilt for my tempted blasphemy.

"There are hundreds, no doubt thousands, of one-legged people out there who feel cheated by the futility of sports participation. I've seen you ski masterfully on one leg, just for fun, while the rest of us watched with humiliation; struggling to be graceful on two. You may've been chosen to help these unfortunates, Pat. They'd listen to you, if you became the best one-legged skier in the world. You could be their inspiration, just as you've been ours for so many years."

Four eyes welled in tears when that conversation ended, and as Pat's car left our driveway, I cursed myself for not being more eloquent. My words felt inadequate. We heard nothing for another two years. I feared the worst.

Pat arrived bearing gifts, when we next saw him—medals he had won from one-legged ski races, newspaper clippings about his victories, and others announcing dinners for the disabled, for which he was guest speaker. Insurance money from the accident had bought him a new car and a 10,000-dollar artificial leg, while earnings from various jobs offered him the opportunity to re-sculpt his nose. Pat even had a girlfriend.

While these stories may seem novelesque in a clinical book about life extension, they are true evidence of psychological victory under fire. Weaker men would have accepted the first psychological insult as a final blow, certain to shorten their life expectancy. By maintaining a portion of the Self separate from roles in society, their importance notwithstanding, both men found new direction and the elusive psychological balance that we should all seek in our quest for healthy longevity. Your life may be thought of as a book: A thick one, comprised of many chapters or merely a paperback pamphlet. Recognize your Self as the author!

Chapter Five

Concluding Remarks

The principal conclusion we hope you have reached is that you can eliminate your middle and your end by beginning (your self-improvement regimen). Your new friend, doctor, and co-author has continued his education in the school of prevention, where he is a perpetual, insatiable student. Mainstream physicians are trained to cure, not to prevent. Dr. Anderson believes in a "holistic" approach to sustaining health in his patients. He also has been trained to cure, but his prescriptions always begin with a sincere doctor/patient dialogue to motivate you towards health and longevity. Your personal history may indicate the need for a diet change, vitamin, mineral, or herb supplementation, antioxidant therapy, hormone replacement, or exercise in lieu of drugs for the discomfort of your condition. He has even employed spiritual guidance in his nurturing progress, having recognized faith as a powerful healing force. He is one of a legion of intelligent physicians, who have recognized a serious void of prevention strategies in the traditional medical school curriculum. These courageous doctors have, on numerous occasions, replaced pharmaceuticals with natural substances that are proven to be effective. Since their preferred, first choice of cure is usually drug-free, these avant-garde doctors have come to be classified as complementary physicians or innovative practitioners of alternative therapies. We predict their domination of the medical profession in the 22nd century.

Mainstream doctors are frightened to challenge the tenets of their powerful watchdog, the AMA, which encourages them to support the generous pharmaceutical establishment, often resulting in drug-dependent patients. Most octogenarians faithfully ingest any product prescribed that promises another day of life, although their miserable condition can hardly be classified as living. Feeble longevity may not be a desirable state for the young, but for the aged who fear death (despite the faith they embrace promising a rapturous after-life), it is better than mortality. Most of these older people cannot see well enough to read the ingredients of a doctor-prescribed medicine. My mom paid 64 dollars for a doctor-prescribed "medicine," which I discovered was no more than a multi-vitamin and mineral capsule. With a magnifying glass, I showed her the label; its list matched the one on my Mega Vita-Min tablets, line for line, though some quantities were higher on my product, which, incidentally, cost only 20 dollars for the same quantity of pills. If this story makes you angry and resentful, you should be. We urge you to rage against medical practitioners like this, who mercilessly prey upon the frailty and devotion of their aged patients. Our grandparents grew up, when it was considered sinful to question authority. They worship doctors to the point of idolatry. "Every day above ground is a good one" is their credo. They will take any drug to ensure another hour, and, they will pay any amount. After all, the "doctor" prescribed it.

We encourage you to question mainstream medical authority, or certainly consider alternative therapy before risking drug-dependency. Evaluation of complementary medicine conjecture does require careful reading, though. The lemmings who blindly take prescribed drugs do not read books like ours. Even this book will raise some doubt in the minds of skeptical readers, and so it should, but *Rage Against Age* is at least backed by photos of an experienced author, who has attained good health and vigor into his 68th year. Your rating of any book should begin with an evaluation of its author. Books are powerful players in the game of self-preservation. Books can shape your value system, fire your faith, change your politics, provide vicarious adventures, and gratify your sexual desires, secret though they may be. As children, we were taught to believe that books in print are infallible words of wisdom for readers who seek the truth. Books, however, also can be subversive, designed to twist your values and reshape them to concur with the beliefs of their authors. The health book industry is no exception. So many conflicting diet books have been published by self-proclaimed nutritionists with no medical background, one must wonder whether they are addressing the same species. Fad diets flood the gossip newspapers, qualified by only one irrelevant prerequisite: The author must be a celebrity. Why would anyone acknowledge their authority for presenting nutritional advice? We live in a gullible society, where the cardinal sin is celebrity idolatry; that is why, many mainstream doctors enjoy exploiting the same kind of idolatry, confident that you will not question their authority. Our book is an honest illustrated record of one man's progress in halting the aging process over a twelve-month period. Consider the following twelve-month progress report, recorded by Dr. Anderson, of his patient and co-author, Frank Covino, as well as his concluding remarks:

Frank is a prime example of what can develop in less than a year from a ketogenic diet, hormone replacement therapy and a sound vitamin, mineral and antioxidant schedule, together with weight-resistance exercise. Some writers would have you believe that such a holistic program is unnecessary if an individual merely balances protein, carbohydrate, and fat consumption. Beware of their agenda and wisely evaluate their credentials. Their conjecture may be designed to sell books. If there was one place which beckoned all of us with a guarantee of health and longevity, we would all be inclined to move to that "zone." Alas, we are all unique, each of us a curious compilation of all our past experiences. We are victims of diet, lifestyle, and the environment in which we were raised. Our habits, behavior, and even our religious preferences have been influenced by the choices of our parents. Few of us are brave enough to break away from early environmental influence; those who do have the courage look to published authors for guidance. The assumption is that publication is justification of the author's authority. Today, self-proclaimed longevity gurus are legion. Book stores are glutted with controversial health and longevity advice, often provided by conflicting, young, innovative "nutritionists" who parrot the opinions of the AMA. Many of these so-called nutritionists have no medical credentials. Whom are we to believe? For two decades doctors have preached the principle cause of obesity to be dietary fat. The strong bones of Ice Age Man belie this concept as clearly as do the lean Eskimos of the Tundra, today, who live to active old ages ingesting caribou, fish, and whale blubber. Many Eskimos have never tasted bread, sugar, or any processed food. Those who do emigrate to towns like Anchorage, adopting the American diet of processed foods, replete with cigarettes, sugar, starch, and liquor are dying before their 70th birthday. Fat phobics, who are choosing sugar-laden processed foods that bear "fat-free" labels are more obese today than when they began their fat-free diet.

Swayed by popular medical conjecture, I, too, have warned my patients about fat ingestion, but principally because fat is a magnet for free radicals. Most of my new patients know nothing about antioxidants. There is also a vast difference between saturated fat, which can certainly clog your arteries, and essential fatty acids, which can clear them. The ingestion of nutritional fats, like olive oil, flaxseed oil, and fish oils like EPA, can trigger your brain to use your own body fat for energy on a ketogenic diet. I believed that years ago, when Dr. Robert Atkins first postulated the theory, but am convinced of it today, because of Frank's transformation in less than a year and because of the energy my wife and I have experienced since adopting the diet ourselves. Compare the "before" photo of Frank at 204 pounds previously presented in Figure 1 with Figure 2, taken recently during one of his workouts. He weighed in this morning at a muscular 185.

The ketogenic diet by no means advocates zero carbohydrates, but merely advises us to discover what our specific tolerance for carbohydrates is, and to not exceed that level, lest the excess be stored as adipose tissue, or, more dangerously, as triglycerides. Moreover, this diet encourages the consumption of complex carbohydrate sources and the omission of, or at least drastic reduction of, simple carbs, like processed sugar "foods" and high-carbohydrate juices. These are your real enemies! Simple carbohydrates cause the highest spikes of insulin. Most overweight people are hyperinsulinemic. Identified as Syndrome X by Dr. Gerald Reaven in 1988, the affliction exacerbates from excessive carbohydrate ingestion, lowering HDL, raising LDL and triglycerides, clots the blood and increases high blood pressure.

Quite simply, we might be a lot healthier if we ate more like our prehistoric ancestors: Any meat, fish, or fowl we can hunt (cooked before it spoils) and any natural plant that is edible but unsweet. Man's health started deteriorating when he began to process foods; it deteriorated more when he imported sugar, and really nose-dived when he began to inject steroids into his cattle and other farm animals to fatten them for profit. Civilization has been a double-edged sword. Sugar is sweet, but it is devastating!

As we have pointed out, there cannot be one diet for everyone, since we are all unique. But we all have a pancreas, and that pancreas will gush insulin, whenever sugar is ingested. Excess insulin will devour your blood sugar, making you feel fatigued. You will reach for more sugar when the crash gets low enough, and the process will continue, until excess triglycerides contribute to the clogging of your arteries and adipose tissue hides your belt. The ketogenic diet is well known to the professional bodybuilding community; they adopt the program three weeks before a contest to deplete their body fat and look more vascular. I thought it would take a year or two for Frank to lose that beer belly, but it was gone in six months. His body fat dropped from 15% to 7%.

You can tell from Frank's "before" photo, that although the beer belly was hideous, the arms and shoulders suggest that he was not unfamiliar with exercise against weight resistance. He had reached a strength plateau, though, with no power or size increases in 15 years. A blood test revealed low testosterone and IGF-I levels. His cholesterol was dangerously elevated at 289, while his triglycerides were nudging 300. After only three months of progressive weight-resistance exercise at higher intensity, daily supplementation of HGH (0.25 cc morning and evening), DHEA, pregnenolone, and tribulus terrestris, plus a doubling of his vitamin, mineral, and antioxidant schedule, his testosterone climbed to 570, his DHEA to 21 from a low 13, and his IGF-1 level tripled. Most gratifying a year later was the lowering of his cholesterol to 184, while his triglycerides sunk 200 points. These last readings have been constant for three months. When creatine was added to his high-protein diet, his strength and energy abounded. The exercise photos corroborate the effectiveness of all the recommendations in our book. When we go to press, Frank will have celebrated his 68th birthday with the power and vitality of a 25-year-old athlete. He is stronger than he has ever been. I have no patient over 50 who can come close to Frank's youthful countenance.

We will not prescribe for our readers. Nor have we offered conjecture without testing our opinions upon ourselves. We do suggest that if a "zone" purports to house the Fountain of Youth, you are going to have to move your body to get there. The complex human organism demands physical activity to function efficiently through its senior years. We also believe (and have proven) that hormone replacement therapy is an exciting modern fuel that can keep our engines revved well beyond a century. (What we have to work on is lowering its cost.) The high number of vitamin, mineral and antioxidant pills that we take daily is still a nuisance. We are working hard to devise encapsulated combinations of nutrients that can lessen the volume of pills. You will hear from us again. Frank was not being facetious when he promised another book from us in 2031. His goal is to be the strongest, most creative centenarian in history. I intend to monitor his progress over the next 32 years, confronting Age with rampant Rage. Stay in touch.

Charles E. Anderson, M.D.

PS Following are a few lab reports, from which you can measure Frank's progress. Especially note the 289 reading of his cholesterol, measured in February of 1996, and its lowering to 190 in April of the same year. Then, look at his cholesterol in February of 1999; it is down to 168.

Laboratory: Quest Diagnostics
Report Date: **02/12/96**
Date of Birth: 10/16/31

Physician: Anderson, Charles M.D.
Patient: Covino, Frank
Age: 64

TEST NAME	RESULT	REFERENCE
Cardiac Panel		
Cholesterol	289 Hi	100-200 mg/dL
Triglycerides	271 Hi	30-175 mg/dL
HDL	49	35-77 mg/dL
LDL	158	62-130 mg/dL
Linear Panel		
Total Protein	7.4	6.0-8.5 g/dL
Albumin	4.5	3.5-5.0 g/dL
Globulin	2.9	2.0-4.0 g/dL
Albumin/Globulin	1.6	1.0-2.0
Alkaline Phosphatase	95	30-159 U/L
LDN	156	60-245 U/L
SGOT	34	0-41 U/L
SGPT	29	0-45 U/L
DHEA	1.3 Lo	1.5-7.0 Ng/mL
PSA	2.0	0-4 Ng/mL

These were the results on Frank's first visit to Dr. Anderson's office. He was started on a natural program and exercise, outlined on page 25 in our text.

Laboratory: Quest Diagnostics
Report Date: **05/06/96**
Date of Birth: 10/16/31

Physician: Anderson, Charles M.D.
Patient: Covino, Frank
Age: 64

TEST NAME	RESULT	REFERENCE
Cardiac Panel		
Cholesterol	190	100-200 mg/dL
Triglycerides	174	30-175 mg/dL
HDL	48	35-77 mg/dL
LDL	121	62-130 mg/dL

The above are Frank's test results after 3 months on a natural program and exercise.

TEST NAME	RESULT	REFERENCE
Thyroid Panel		
T3	30	25-36%
T4	5	4.5-12.0 ug/dL
FTI	1.9	1.4-3.7
TSH (Thyroid Stimulation Hormone from pituitary gland.)	5.8 Hi	0.3-5.0 uLU/mL

Frank was started on Armour Thyroid ¼ grain daily as the elevated TSH showed the need for thyroid supplementation.

Laboratory: Quest Diagnostics
Report Date: **06/09/97**
Date of Birth: 10/16/31

Physician: Anderson, Charles M.D.
Patient: Covino, Frank
Age: 65

TEST NAME	RESULT	REFERENCE
Cardiac Panel		
Cholesterol	193	100-200 mg/dL
Triglycerides	171	30-200 mg/dL
HDL	42	35-77 mg/dL
LDL	117	62-130 mg/dL
TSH	2.8	.3-5.0 uLU/mL
DHEA	1.4 Lo	1.5-7.0 Ng/mL
Testosterone	81 Lo	280-1100 Ng/dL
TSH	2.8	.3-5.0 uLU/mL

At this point, Frank was started on DHEA 50 mg daily and Testosterone Cream 50 mg/gram 3 times a week. Also, he was to continue his Armour Thyroid ¼ grain daily.

Laboratory: Quest Diagnostics
Report Date: **05/29/98**
Date of Birth: 10/16/31

Physician: Anderson, Charles M.D.
Patient: Covino, Frank
Age: 66

TEST NAME	RESULT	REFERENCE
Cardiac Panel		
Cholesterol	184	100-200 mg/dL
Triglycerides	138	30-200 mg/dL
HDL	44	35-77 mg/dL
LDL	104	62-130 mg/dL
PSA	3.9	0.4
DHEA	2.0	1.5-7.0 Ng/mL
Testosterone	254	241-827 Ng/dL
IGF-1 (Measures Human Growth Hormone)	108	71-290
TSH	2.8	0.3-5.0
Liver Panel	Within normal limits	

At this point Frank was started on Human Growth Hormone. He was continuing on DHEA, Testosterone Cream and Armour Thyroid.

Laboratory: Quest Diagnostics
Report Date: **02/19/99**
Date of Birth: 10/16/31

Physician: Anderson, Charles M.D.
Patient: Covino, Frank
Age: 67

TEST NAME	RESULT	REFERENCE
Cardiac Panel		
Cholesterol	168	100-200 mg/dL
Triglycerides	112	30-200 mg/dL
HDL	42	35-77 mg/dL
LDL	104	62-130 mg/dL
DHEA	2.3	1.5-7.0 Ng/mL
IGF-1 (Measures Human Growth Hormone)	191	71-290
TSH	2.5	0.3-5
Testosterone	288	241-327 Ng/dL

At this point, Frank was to continue HGH (Human Growth Hormone), Testosterone, Armour Thyroid and DHEA.

We are authors who practice what we preach. We have recommended no diet or micro-nutrient supplement that we have not tested on ourselves. We have read many books, tested many supplements, and have tried various workout protocols to qualify our guidance. We have not merely presented evidence; we are the evidence, and we invite your inspection, if you hold any doubt that strength and health can improve with age, rather than decline.

Assuming this enormous task of documenting our discoveries, our long quest for the Fountain of Youth, is a calculated risk. Disapproval is the nightmare of any author. Dr. Anderson's curriculum vitae, along with 25 years in private practice, and my strong mental and physical countenance, as I begin my 68th year, should be sufficient credentials to grant us the right to publish our rejuvenation conjecture. We expect disapproval from the mainstream medical community, many of whom feel that vitamins do no more than create rich urine. We anticipate a vitriolic response from the Florida Chamber of Commerce for deprecating the lethargic shuffling dead of Collins Avenue, who never miss a day noshing a pastry at Wolfie's. We expect to hear loud responses from the dedicated sports spectators for attacking the Little League syndrome as a form of child abuse, devastating to children who do not make the team. We will probably be rejected by red-neck homophobics for defining same-sex preference as often the preordained result of hormonal imbalance, a mistake of nature, rather than a perversity. And, we are certain that flak will be fired by some fundamental religious communities for our stand on the personal moral choice of divorce from abusive relationships to protect the psyche and open a door to a new life. We have placed our reputations "on the line" in presenting what we firmly believe to be the truth. The ball is now in your court.

Let us assume that our book has alerted you to health-securing options you may never have considered. In your new quest for active longevity, where do you begin? What tests constitute your initial step? Your first volley should be to schedule a thorough blood and urine analysis.

From the former, you can learn whether you are deficient in DHEA, pregnenolone, free testosterone, estrogen and IGF-1. Your PSA, thyroid and dehydroxytestosterone levels also can be measured, as can your triglyceride and cholesterol count, HDL and LDL. The diagnostic report returned from your blood will include a reference list of ranges that are "normal." You may then compare your levels with these, to determine your deficiencies. Work with an alternative doctor who knows natural drug equivalents. Your complementary physician can recommend ameliorative dosages of corresponding supplements.

Supplementation can not only raise your blood levels to normal range; it can boost them to youthful levels and significantly stall the aging process. Drugs should be a last resort.

Of course, no test will be meaningful if administered by a doctor who keeps the analysis and prognosis to himself. Too many physicians live in an ivory tower. Ego-inflated with the knowledge their years of study have provided, many refuse to have diagnostic conversation with their less-educated patients. You have a right to know what caused your condition, whether there are drug-free alternatives that may cure it and what sidc effects are known to follow the ingestion of any drugs they may prescribe. In layman's language, thank you. Dr. Harvard may have graduated summa cum laude, but his "bedside manner" may be as deficient as his penmanship. Your relationship with your doctor should be high on your list of importance, as it can either prolong your life or accelerate your obituary.

A schedule of effective supplements' prerequisite is proper diet and weight-resistant exercise. Although your blood type and activity level can affect the quantity and type of food that you should eat, there are some adjustments that can help everyone stall the aging process. If we were your personal trainers we would advise you to:

1. Eliminate, or at least minimize, sugar and starchy foods.
2. Minimize or eliminate gluten products. If you must eat bread, make it occasional, and only choose multi-grain products.
3. Eliminate or minimize dairy products. If you must ingest milk, make it skim or 1% fat. Trash all processed cheeses. If you must eat cheese, find the hardest variety, like Locatelli, Romano, Asiago, or Parmesan.
4. Upgrade your protein. The purest, of highest biological value is cross-filtered ionized whey, in the form of protein powder, available at any good health store. Fish is the second choice. Increase your seafood ingestion. Lean meat is next, with minimum fat content. Then, chicken, preferably without skin. Beans and legumes can satisfy the protein needs of vegetarians, but plant protein is not as complete as meat protein. If you are smart enough to exercise, ingest one gram of protein for every pound of your body weight. Just do not ingest more than 45 mg at one time. Despite what you may have read, cooked eggs offer good protein and HAVE NEVER BEEN PROVEN TO RAISE CHOLESTEROL levels. Lecithin in the yolk of an egg is sufficient to emulsify its cholesterol content. The egg is a perfect food.

Frank lowered his cholesterol from 287 to 165 while ingesting a dozen eggs per week.

5. Buy a juicer and begin every day with a vegetable juice, predominantly green, for the chlorophyll will detox your digestive system. Drink two or three glasses a day, if you can. Micro-minimize sugar juices, though; some carry twice as many carbs as the fruit that produced them.
6. Drink water often, even if you feel you are not thirsty. Try for at least ten glasses a day.
7. Discover your carbohydrate tolerance level with Ketostix, as we recommended, and don't exceed it. Excess simple carbohydrates are a primary source of body fat and high triglycerides. Green vegetables and some low carbohydrate fruit are your best choices.
8. Eat more often, but smaller food quantities. Five to six times a day is a good regimen with no carbohydrates after 8 PM. Try to ingest most of your carbohydrates at breakfast and within two hours of heavy exercise.
9. Eat more oats, proven to lower cholesterol levels and also provide necessary fiber. Cereals and some high-grain breads offer a sufficient amount, if you would rather not take oats via capsule supplement.
10. Begin an exercise program and recognize physical culture as the catalyst, without which, all your supplements and diet modifications have been fruitless and in vain.
11. Have your hormone level checked and restored to youthful parameters, if they are low.
12. Begin an antioxidant supplementation schedule; start by considering those that we take along with your vitamin and mineral preferences.
13. Add creatine, glutamine, HMB, alpha-lipoic acid, and phosphatidyl serine to your daily diet.
14. Cross-train by including some sport along with your weight training.
15. Monitor your progress by consulting with a qualified complementary physician, preferably one who practices what he preaches.

No longer a fruitless quest, active longevity is now attainable, and human life expectancy will be lengthened in the 21st century, as more books like *Rage Against Age* are published. Hormone Replacement Therapy will be a major player. Exercise will become as perfunctory as tooth brushing. HGH will be recognized as the true Fountain of Youth. Presently, destructive digestion acids would destroy any orally administered HGH, before it found its way to your blood stream. Affluent celebrities have clung to their youth by periodically injecting Human Growth Hormone, from recombinant products like Humatrope, but the average reader could not afford the cost, and most of you fear injections. We predict new pathways to be introduced in the 21st century, like nasal spray transporters, which would be less costly and more acceptable by the needle-shy public. We predict the lifting of bans against medically prescribed ergogenic supplements ingested by Olympic athletes, who will then shatter the phenomenal records set during our time. The professional bodybuilding community, eager to develop the most powerful, massive male form, will continue to lose participants from the injection of excessive steroid substances and diuretics, until one of their families hires a good lawyer to sue their promoters, as the cigarette companies are currently being sued, for criminal disregard of health standards and the creation of drug-dependent champions. These litigations will arouse new interest in natural physique development that is still strong, but healthy, and certainly more symmetrical. Bodybuilding gurus and ergogenic scientists will continue to be watched by the medical community, which has been reluctant to try human experimentation, for bodybuilders' latest strategies that promote strength, endurance, and active longevity. Natural pro-hormones, like 19-Norandrostenediol, will replace illegal steroids like Deca-Durabolin, producing vital strength steroids, like nandrolone, in the liver.

Cancer has been the big killer of our century, strengthened by fools who smoke and by the fumes of industrial pollution. We predict and encourage a national ban, which will make the U.S. the first country to be smoke-free. Addicts, intolerant of the infringement upon their "rights," will leave the country, probably to Canada, hopefully to the moon. Smoking will continue to proliferate in Europe and throughout the Asian community, and cancer will concomitantly rise there.

Telomerase technology will finally defeat cancer, spearheaded by such companies as the forerunner, Geron. Telomeres may be another key player in preventing age-related diseases. Telomeres are repeated sequences of DNA, found at chromosome endings; they break down with cell division, shortening each time a cell divides. When their length shortens to a specific size, cell division stops and the cell becomes senescent, expressing genes aberrationally. Some genes formerly expressed by young cells are turned off. This process of imbalance causes mutations that activate oncogenes and shut off tumor suppressant genes, giving birth to a pre-cancerous cell.

Curiously, the telomerase activated by the attachment of a telomere to a precancerous cell gives the killer cell immortality, until the host recipient dies. Telomerase is found in only a few normal cells, like reproductive cells, probably responsible for genetic code inheritance from one generation to another; it is a germ-like enzyme comprised of RNA (ribonucleic acid) and a series of proteins.

Geron is trying to develop a telomerase suppresser, which will take life away from telomeres that are attached to cancerous cells. What should logically follow that development, probably close to the turn of the century, is technology that will transfer telomerase back to senescent cells, rejuvenating them with nature's most basic source of energy. This development can, and probably will, extend the life span of man significantly, especially if he adopts the life style recommended in this book. *Rage Against Age* will be the audible cry of 21st century health-hungry inhabitants. Your children will be witnesses. Alert them now! Other companies feverishly studying cell aging and immortality at this time include Chiron and Lark Technologies.

Most frightening to the authors, since we lack psychological credentials, was the task of addressing psychological imbalances and stresses of our daily lives, and what we feel is necessary to overcome these obstacles. Mental stress can be as significant as physical neglect or abuse in accelerating the aging process. Some of us, because of life's commitments, have had "no time" to examine our pain.

There is no magic bullet for defending against psychological trauma. We are, of course, all different, but Frank's concept of Self-powered galaxies can help you to overcome painful trauma, if you learn to apply it. First, you must be motivated. To cure the illnesses that are spawned from our exposure to unexpected traumatic events, we must begin with an enthusiastic approach to life, and expect future events to be unpredictable. With a positive attitude, we must confront all challenges, respond, and move on to new adventures. Support from family and friends is helpful, of course, but you must be prepared for lack of support from them also, as even they are but planets, albeit close in orbit to your Self. The survival of your Self must never be totally dependent on any one of them. Your future is in your own hands. Success is within your reach, if you truly believe it achievable.

Whether you will profit from exposure to another human's experiences is, of course, not assured. You will, however, be affected by it one way or another. We all are the sum of that to which we have been exposed: People, books, music, art, drama, war. Our book is but one small stimulus in the complex development of your Self. We hope it will encourage you to make of your life a vast galaxy of vital experience. The book is your fuel. Rage will start your engine. You can regain and sustain the energy, strength, and vitality of youth.

Rage Against Age has been offered with the hope of inspiring readers to take charge of themselves, to develop their physical, mental and spiritual potential close to their inherited capacity. The futile inevitability of mortality gives us two choices. One choice is to selfishly languish in a perpetual state of hedonism, motivated by instant gratification, tolerate years of illness and pain from lethargy and lack of health education, die after six decades, leaving nothing behind except children (doomed to follow our example) and accumulated possessions. A second choice is to investigate our nature, strengthen our bodies and minds, remain active and creative well beyond the sixth decade, leaving a few significant marks behind (besides babies) that may elevate us above the level of animals and may justify our existence. Those "marks" need not be great works of art or voluminous books; they could be a few warm sweaters or knitted socks, a hand-built home, planted perennial gardens, trees from seed sown by you—creative marks that elevate us above the level of lesser brained animals. Other marks of immortality could be born from the simple act of touching others of our species, to help them rise above the level of primitive existence, the way teachers touch minds or missionaries touch souls. If mortality must be inevitable, the only tangible defense we have against that terrifying sentence is to leave a part of us behind.

You really can take charge. You can learn more about caring for yourself from books like ours. You can develop a countenance that will be respected not merely by your peer group, but one that your children will admire and possibly look forward to developing themselves. The bonus from attaining active health and longevity is that the doors for productivity and adventure will remain open for you well beyond your sixth decade. When your final breath comes, you will pass peacefully with a smile, knowing that you have indeed left a few marks, that you have seen more, visited more places and lived more than your primitive provincial neighbor. Moreover, if you truly believe in the "resurrection of the body," you will proudly present yours as one that has been developed to its fullest potential, intellect notwithstanding.

You are fortunate enough to live in an age where it is even possible to correct Nature's insults, as you move toward the development of the most perfect you. For the myopic, there are contact lenses; hearing aids for the audibly impaired become more effective and unobtrusive every year; artificial limbs have become more manipulative; plastic surgery can remodel faces wrinkled from stress and excessive sun exposure, and silicone can fill breasts drained and flattened by thirsty suckling; liposuction can accelerate the re-sculpting of your body if you are too impatient to try it naturally by exercise and proper diet restrictions. Feel old and you will become old very rapidly. Think old and you will become old. You are your thoughts; so think young and you will remain youthful. Why not rage against nature's insults? Why shouldn't we do all we can to retain active health and longevity? You have but one life. You can waste it or you can take charge now and become the most healthy and attractive you that is naturally possible. This book is your survival manual. We will close it with an insightful thought from the poet Robert Browning:

> "Grow old, along with me!
> The best is yet to be,
> The last of life, for which the first was made."

—Rabbi Ben Ezra [1864]
— Robert Browning (1812-1898)

Textual List of Figures

From full extension, with the back of your hand facing forward, slowly curl the weight upward, twisting your hand when the forearm parallels the floor. Raise the pinky higher than the thumb for maximum biceps contraction.

Twist the hand again, as you press the weight overhead, to end with the palm of your hand forward. This twist involves more deltoid fibers.

The prefix "bi" refers to the split of the biceps. Its function is to contract or "curl" the fist to the shoulder; this is the cable variation. Use one hand for more intense concentration.

Two-arm curl on a Scott bench may be varied by changing from a close grip of the bar to a wide grip. The former variation stresses the inside fibers, while a wide grip is better for outside biceps development.

Two-arm variation of the "French" curl. Start with the elbows close to your ears.

Fully extended, with the elbows stationary. Perform your repetitions slowly There is no better triceps exercise than the "French" curl.

Hammer Curl, completed. Perform these curls slowly. For a greater amount of time under tension, try "one and a halves" (a full curl immediately followed by a half curl). Alternate arms, of course, and keep the elbow stationary.

Two-arm Triceps Press Down. Keep the elbows stationary and the movement slow. Note the characteristic "horseshoe" shape of Frank's triceps.

One-arm variation of the Triceps Press Down. The elbow must not move.

The Wrist Curl, start position. Let the bar drop to your fingertips.

Finish position of the Wrist Curl contracts the Palmaris. Compare this muscle with the gastrocnemius (calf) muscles of the lower leg. The muscles of the legs duplicate those of the arms.

Fully contracted Leg Curl. Hold the tension for a count or two, before returning to the start position.

Hold the contraction for a count or two, before lowering the weight back to the start position. Leg extensions develop the quadriceps of the thighs, like the French curls

Appendix

Following is a list of vitamin companies and medical compounding pharmacies with whom Dr. Anderson has worked with over the years. He has great confidence in their products.

Da Vinci Laboratories of Vermont
20 New England Drive
Essex Junction, VT 05453-1504
(800) 325-1776
In Canada (800) 510-3676

Food Science of Vermont
20 New England Drive C-1504
Essex Junction, VT 05453-1504
(800) 874-9444

Douglas Laboratories
600 Boyce Road
Pittsburgh, PA 15205
(800) 245-4400
Special thanks to Carol Gardner for assisting us for many years.

GeroVita/Medi-Plex
520 Washington Street
Marina del Rey, CA 90292
(800) 292-6006

Pure Encapsulation
490 Boston Post Road
Sudbury, MA 017766
(800) 753-2277

Kelley Pharmacy
Scott Brown, Owner/Pharmacist
Timber Lane Medical Complex
Kennedy Drive
South Burlington, VT 05403
(802) 862-6855

Medaus Compounding Pharmacy
Steven Russell, Owner/Pharmacist
2524 Valleydale Road, Suite 100
Birmingham, AL 35244

Medical Center Pharmacy
Richard Farr, Owner/Pharmacist
3675 So. Rainbow Blvd.
Las Vegas, NV 89103
(800) 723-7455

We also advise our readers to consider monthly publications or newsletters, as the field of medicine and physical culture is changing so rapidly. These publications are mandatory to stay informed in this ever-changing arena. Here are a few:

Journal of Longevity
Published by Health Quest Publications
316 California Avenue
Reno, NV 89509
Glenn Braswell, Publisher
Rob Tepper, Editor
Beverly Berwald, Managing Editor (who has been a great help to Dr. Anderson over the years)

Health and Healing
Published by Phillips, Inc.
7811 Montrose Road
Potomac, MD 20854-3394
(800) 539-8219
Dr. Julian Whitaker, Editor

The following magazines offer the latest information and accessibility of pro-hormones, plus professional guidance and exposure to the latest bodybuilding strategies, primarily for men:

Ironman Magazine
1 (800)-570-IRON (ext. 2)

MuscleMag International
6465 Airport Road
Mississauga, Ontario
Canada, L4V 1E4.

Pump Magazine
1 (800) 899-8157

Highly recommended for women is the magazine *Oxygen*. Call 1 (905) 678-7311 to subscribe.

Spearheading the contemporary movement against steroid supplementation and promoting nature body development is the magazine *Muscle Media 2000*. Call 1 (800) 297-9776, Dept. 3222 for a subscription. Bill Phillips' courageous stand against drug abuse has effectively cleaned up the bodybuilding industry

Older publication houses like the empire of Joe Weider continue to inspire us with magazines like *Muscle and Fitness*, *Flex* and *Shape* (for women), but be advised that the gargantuan bodies of the body builders from Joe's stables can only be built with the help of anabolic steroids and dangerous diuretics that are illegal drugs as classified by the U.S. FDA. Competitors of the Weider-sponsored Mr. Olympia contest are frustrated with the knowledge that they have no chance of attaining recognition without getting locked into an unnatural anabolic steroid, diuretic and estrogen-blocking supplement schedule. Proof that their massive sizes (some weighing in at 300 pounds) are drug-induced is evidenced by how rapidly these champions shrink when they are forced to stop injecting because of life-threatening side effects. We predict that even Joe Weider, once a natural participant in the healthy sport of bodybuilding, will recognize the potential damage to young enthusiasts that emphasis upon superhuman mass as a qualification of Mr. Olympia status has, particularly with the acceptance of the Olympic committee of natural bodybuilding as an International event, subject to drug testing.

Please support your local health food stores. However, if you cannot find this book, you can order it directly from the publisher or from one of the authors, if you would like a signed edition. Call for lower bulk-quantity rates.

Health food stores that have been very helpful in our area:

Vites & Herb
Williston & Middlebury, VT

Healthy Living
South Burlington, VT

Moon Meadow
South Burlington, VT

Purple Shutter
Burlington, VT

GNC—across the nation, General Nutrition Centers dot every major city. Look for the closest in your yellow pages.

ORDER FORM

New Century Promotions
3711 Alta Loma Drive
Bonita, CA 91902
(800) 768-8484

Please send ______ copy(copies) of Rage Against Age at $21.95 per copy.

Limited signed editions are available from either author:

Frank Covino
Waitsfield, VT 05673-0420, Dept. R.

Dr. Charles Anderson
175 Pearl Street
Essex Junction, VT 05452, Dept. R.

Please send ______ signed copy(copies) of Rage Against Age at $25.00 per copy. Shipping: Book Rate. $3.00 for the first copy and $1.50 for each additional copy.

Ship To:

Name________________________________
Address______________________________
City________________________State______Zip_____________

☐ Check or Money Order for autographed copies.
☐ Check or Credit Card for publishers orders only.
☐ Discover ☐ Visa ☐ MasterCard ☐ American Express
Card Number____________________Exp. Date_____________

Signature____________________________

Give the gift that keeps on giving – *Rage Against Age.*